A Glass Glued with Gold

Heather Nisbet

Copyright © Heather Nisbet 2024

All rights reserved. The author asserts their moral right under the Copyright, Designs and Patents Act 1988 to be identified as the author of this work.

Published by Golden Glue Publishing.

Except for the quotation of small passages for the purposes of criticism and review, no part of this publication may be reproduced, stored in a retrieval system, or transmitted, in any form or by any means, electronic, mechanical, photocopying, recording or otherwise, except under the terms of the Copyright, Designs and Patent Act 1988 without the prior consent of the publisher above.

ISBN: 978-1-0686957-3-5

Friends are the family we choose.

This book is gratefully dedicated to every member of my family, biological and chosen. Thank you to each person who has been a part of my journey. You are my source of strength, my memory-makers and so much more besides. I love and appreciate you more than you'll ever know. There aren't enough words in the world or time left in my life to express how much I have needed you and how unconditionally you've always been there. You know who you are and you mean everything to me. My heart—full of love, my endless thanks, and this book, are for you.

Jenna, you are the sister I got to choose and the 'daughter' I never knew I looked old enough to have! You have made my life better and this book possible. Thank you is not enough, but you are, as you always have been. Keep shining.

Contents

Introduction

Do you know who you are?
The miracle is you.................................. 1
You and I.. 9
Mirror, mirror....................................... 29
Breathe... 47

Do you know what has happened to you?
Time wears a white coat........................... 59
Labels... 75
Your shoes don't define you; it's the way
that you wear them 93
The black dog's bark............................... 105
The hero behind the mask........................ 123
Never pick a petal or two......................... 135

Do you want to live this way?
Non piangere perché una cosa finisce,
sorridi perché é accaduta......................... 155
Enough is enough.................................. 168
Tape and glue and cracks of gold............... 177

Mental health support services.................. 193
Dear reader.. 200
Acknowledgements................................. 203
References... 207

Introduction

Do you know who you are?
Do you know what has happened to you?
Do you want to live this way?

These three questions formed the premise of a season 10 episode of Grey's Anatomy in 2014. It was based on a deeply profound, in my case at least, 'sliding doors' type of story. Narrating the episode, the character of Cristina Yang asked the above questions to a critically-ill patient, whose ventilator was about to be removed. Watching that episode for the first time, and during every viewing since, it felt like Sandra Oh was speaking directly to me. I've contemplated the deeply personal—and, at times, painful—answers about myself and my own life ever since.

Those questions motivated me to write this book. I wanted—needed, even—to explore the answers and their implications for my past, present, and perhaps, most significantly, my future. It was whilst planning and penning this content that I began to wonder: how would other people answer these same questions? Would it be too much to hope that we could begin to love ourselves and others just a little more if we got to know ourselves a little better?

Could this book enable us to more acutely understand the pain that strengthens us and the decisions and experiences that shape us?

I often pass people on a journey; I share the same space or moment in time with them, and I wonder what their story is. I imagine who they are, how they're feeling, and what their life is really like beneath the surface. It's all too easy to assume—especially if we know the person and have some of this information already. But the final picture may be nothing more than our own perception, a Magic Eye illusion of who they are, based on who we think we see. I think we do this with ourselves, too. We construct our self-image based on what we interpret from our reflection, from our interactions, from what's said and done to us. In turn, this domino-effect often determines and drives what we say and do to ourselves. Rather than it being self-indulgent to ask ourselves these questions, it's necessary for us to understand where we've come from, what we have survived, the people and events that have impacted us and who we are as a result.

We all keep chapters of ourselves to ourselves. There are those that are too painful or poignant to read aloud, which are buried so deeply beneath the surface that we may underestimate their significance. Maybe the same is true for you. You are so much more than what anyone sees in you. I believe that we're all so much more than we see in ourselves. We need to take the time to look, to understand, to accept, to love—and maybe, to even forgive the person that lies beneath it all.

I wrote this book after realising the importance of respecting and nurturing the relationship we have with ourselves. I forced myself to take the time to understand how our past bleeds into the present and how it flows into our future. As a result of this introspection, I finally acknowledged that it's okay not to be okay, so long as we're never 'not okay' alone. More than once, life has brought me to my knees, but against all the odds, I didn't stay there. I would love this book to serve as an outstretched hand that helps you get back on your feet again.

I acknowledge that my story will not look like yours. The reason I'm sharing my experiences is to demonstrate that my suggestions and support come from a place of love. They're borne from a lived experience that almost broke me in ways I never expected to recover from. On reflection, they gave me a strength I never knew I possessed. All along, this strength was my buried superpower. I'm sharing my experiences because I survived what I never expected to, and I desperately want the same outcome for you. Our pain, traumas, and experiences are not to be compared to or ranked against anyone else's. Hopefully, they can instead become tools and strategies others use when they feel at their lowest or most vulnerable.

Whatever you take from reading this, I hope it includes enjoyment, a deeper appreciation of yourself, and the tools to nurture and sustain your mental health. I hope you take away the knowledge that whatever has or is happening to you, you're important. You and your story matter. You're not alone. You're abundantly enough.

All it takes is one person, one moment, one decision, to change your life forever. To change your perspective, so that you reimagine your dreams, your purpose, and your potential. To force you to reevaluate everything you think you know, want and believe. To help you achieve, and to encourage you to ask yourself the toughest, most painful of questions.
Do you know who you are?
Do you understand what has happened to you?
Do you want to live this way?
What would your answers be?

To every single person who's investing in themselves and reading this book, thank you so much. In all honesty, sharing this book with you means more to me than you could ever realise, and I hope that whatever you take from it, it's positive, and it helps you make peace with every piece of yourself and your story.

Heather x

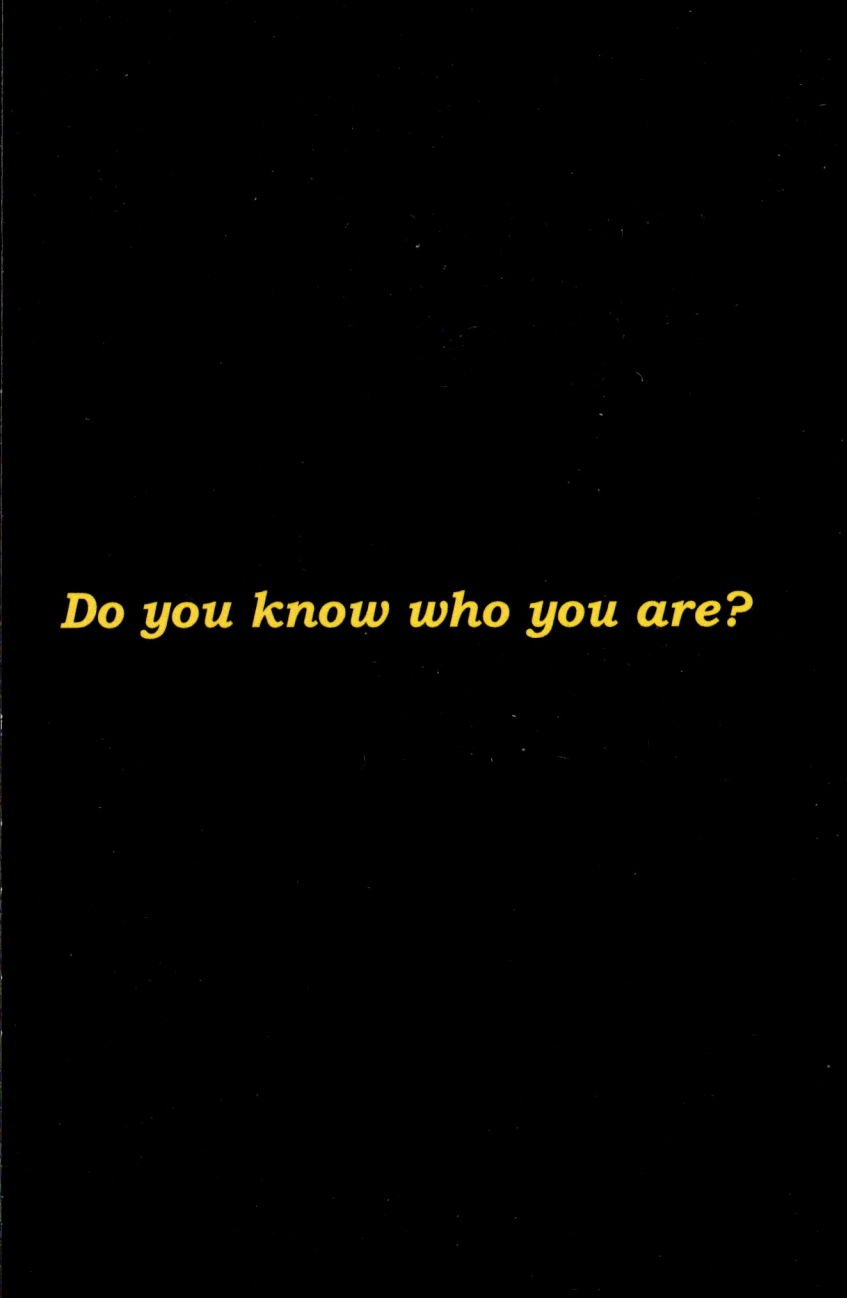

Do you know who you are?

The miracle is you

Life can cause us to feel broken for any number of reasons. It can happen over a prolonged period of time or in a moment that blindsides us. Like a stone cast into open water, the situation may only skim the surface and yet leave a ripple effect of consequences in its wake before sinking out of sight, forever weighing heavy in the depths of the heart and mind. Regardless of the source of your pain or situation, you are not the problem. You're a person in need of love, support, coping strategies, and positive outcomes. The fact you're here—that you continue to be here—is a miracle.

If there comes a point in your life when you feel unable to see beyond your current situation or emotional reactions, please know you're not alone. I hope this letter gives you a different perspective. I hope it brings you some clarity and peace. I hope these words can be a friend to you, and that they will sit alongside you in quiet reassurance of your worth.

Dear you,
A miracle is defined as 'an extraordinary and remarkable event or development that brings very welcome consequences'.

I can't comment on how extraordinary and remarkable your arrival into this world was, but it's probably safe to say that it wasn't an especially glamorous entrance. I think we all have that much in common. Your life, its starting point, and the ensuing years, are utterly unique. In fact, you put the 'you' in 'unique'. You are the irreplaceable and miraculous consequence of that momentous moment, which should never be underestimated or apologised for. A mould was cast in the shape of you, which can never be repeated.

Let's put this into context. Data from the United Nations suggests that there were eight billion people inhabiting Earth in 2022. This figure is rising on a daily basis. Eight billion people with eight billion individual identities and eight billion sets of experiences. Eight billion human journeys, each as different and valuable as the next. You are amongst them. You may be just one person, but you're as rare and worthy as any other person who leaves a set of footprints on this planet. You're as capable, as important, as full of potential, and as perfectly imperfect as the person who walks behind, beside, and ahead of you. You are miraculous, because against all odds and challenges, you exist, adapt, and survive. You are a miracle. Whatever life may tell you to the contrary, you're the welcome consequence of whatever led you to be here. You're the positive spark that punctuates the darkness, that forces breath into the world, that leaves a mark and makes a difference. You are the difference. You may be one of eight billion people walking this planet, but no one other than you will ever walk in your shoes. No one will tell your story or feel your losses, your lowest ebbs or your highest elations as you will—and that is your miraculous superpower. You're here for a reason, and you get to decide what that reason is.

Live each day as if it were on purpose, just as you are. There are eight billion people in the world, a truly inconceivable quantity. The fact that you're one of them isn't a design fault, something to offer an apology for or a problem to be rectified—it's a miracle to be celebrated.

Even on your worst day, during your lowest point, you matter, and your light still shines. The world needs your light.
If you're:
- *drowning in impossible choices*
- *facing insurmountable challenges*
- *blinded by panic*
- *overcome by fear*
- *choking on bitter resentment*
- *consumed by grief*
- *scared*

- *lonely*
- *anxious*
- *lost or emotionally empty*

...you are worth the effort to be repaired from the inside out, however broken you may feel.

This is not the end of your story.

Your shell—the superficial exterior the world sees and judges you on—is irrelevant. It's a part of you, but it's not what matters or what defines you. Imagine you're looking at yourself in a full-length mirror. Your naked body is covered in post-it notes, each one bearing a label, a description, a guise of who you are. You're clothed in the definitions you've worn for a lifetime that have become your second skin. Some describe all that you think you are, whilst others describe all that you believe you're not.

You wear the following as your trademark, your unapologetic apology to an unforgiving world and as your cross to bear:

- *your racial origin*
- *your level of education*
- *your religious conviction*
- *your marital status*
- *your fertility*
- *your employment status*
- *your sexual orientation*
- *your recognised or preferred gender identity*
- *your shoe size*
- *your BMI*

The miracle is you

- *your height*
- *your medical conditions, ailments and afflictions*
- *your bank balance*
- *your sexual history*
- *your deepest regrets*
- *your biggest fears*
- *your talents*

The title of every role you fulfil in life, every hat you wear, every part you play. Your broken promises, missed opportunities and shattered dreams, your visible scars, disfigurements, and disabilities—and the invisible ones, too.

Your phone, National Insurance, and house numbers are a part of your identity, but they're not identifiers of who you are. They tell others nothing of note or substance about you, what you've lived through and all that you have to give. The same is true for the number of years you've been alive and the number you see when you look at the dial on the scales or the label in your clothes.

Each label overlaps the next; each one as stifling as a noose around your neck.

Now imagine you remove these post-it notes. You pull one mark-inducing label at a time until your naked skin is raw, with only one label remaining. This one cannot be removed: **human**. *Imagine if each of the eight billion people around* *the globe were to do the same, in some silent, simultaneous undressing of all that life has given them to wear. For as different and unique as we are, we're each no more or less worthy than the person we compare ourselves to. Every other person is as flawed and as fallible as we are, including those who would have us believe otherwise.*

You're at your most vulnerable when you're naked, and yet you're also at your most whole.

You're not a stereotype. You're not a victim. You're not a disappointment. You're not a failure. You're not a collection of adjectives, a problem to be solved or something to be fixed. You're making your way through a life that doesn't come with a rewind function, a pause button, a chance to skip forward to the highlights or the ability to start over from the beginning. Take a moment to consider what extraordinary and remarkable strength it takes you to get through your most difficult days. Contemplate what a significant difference you make to the people in your life, all labels aside, without you even realising it. Your journey hasn't been easy, but you're here and you're trying and that is, in my opinion, everything. The world will not always see you as you deserve to be seen. It will not always bring you to your feet when you're on your knees; it will not always lead you to hope when you're lost, nor strengthen you when you're at your most vulnerable. Unlike you, the world is not enough.

The James Bond franchise may have brought this concept to our attention, but the problem goes back further than Ian Fleming's imagination. It's deeper than villainy, espionage, and subterfuge. It has human animosity, indifference, and intolerance at its core. The world is not patient, loving, tolerant, forgiving or wise enough, and this is the biggest threat to our internal and external relationships. It's possibly even the poison that determines our survival. It feels as though it's getting harder to distinguish where the opinions of the world end and our own perceptions start. Social media makes the opinions of others more accessible; however, they can drown out our own thoughts whilst masquerading as the truth.

Please believe me when I say that no one knows you better than you know yourself. No one's opinion of you should speak more loudly than your opinion of you, unless they're providing light to counteract your darkness. Think of your life as the most precious, remarkable thing you will ever own, and be selective over who has access to it. The world is not always brave enough to accept the change you bring; it may not seem grateful enough to recognise the contribution you make, nor appear perceptive enough to see the strength behind your struggles. It's not always wise enough to appreciate that we're all miracles within the mundane. Don't let the world silence your voice, define your worth or decide your path and potential. Do not give it permission to harden your soul, to make you small or stop you from being your biggest cheerleader and advocate.

Perfection is the unachievable and inconsistent goalpost that we shackle ourselves to in the hope it will set us free. Our freedom comes from the acknowledgement of our imperfections. It comes from our belief in the strength we have to move forward, from one soul-destroying and strength-affirming moment to the next. Freedom is the ability to rise above the noise, to see through the doubt and to believe that we're as unique and miraculous as we were born to be. We haven't got it all figured out yet, but the journey isn't over yet. We have the gift of time. So long as we continue to give ourselves another tomorrow, we give ourselves the permission to keep trying, to keep healing and moving forward, and that's one of the greatest gifts there is.

For all of these reasons, and countless more besides—the miracle is you.

You and I

*I reflect on you
with introspection,
remembering
a lost direction.
There is no judgement,
how could there be?
For I am you
and you are me.*

*I was there for
the first step you took;
I held your pen
as you wrote your book.
You closed your eyes
and I could see
you walking on
with dignity.
I know your story
etched line by line
across your face
by the hands of time.*

*They see the cover
concealing the plot.
They see so little
whilst we see the lot.
I recognise those*

precious eyes with pride.
I've felt their pain
each time you cried.
I've known the humour
of each laughter line.
They map our journey,
they let the light shine
through. Yet you obscure
your light, you mask your pain.
You hide that part of you,
time and again.

For those you love
you are their tree;
rooted, steadfast, with a heart
of integrity.
But do not settle
where your roots are planted.
Breathe in the moment.
Follow the life you wanted.

You overcame each challenge
you never knew you could.
You survived the pain
you never thought you would.
They won't all like you,
but don't you see?
They are not the ones
who will set you free.

*They do not know you
and those that do,
well, they, like me,
would give the world for you.*

*You must believe
you are worth the fight.
Take back your voice.
Take back your light.
This is our story,
my promise to you.
For you are me
and I am you.*

Fears and phobias can be companions to us all at some point in our lives. The dark has never really bothered me, and yet it was whilst lying alone one night in the dark in April 2015, that the most terrifying experience of my life occurred. As tears soaked my cheeks, emptying my body of all my emotions and sense of worth and purpose, I felt the sensation of my heart breaking. Even though I'd never experienced a feeling like it before in my life, in that moment, time stopped, and I knew instantly what was happening.

I'd read about broken heart syndrome as an abstract but very real medical condition; this was my experience of it. I felt as though I couldn't breathe. In that moment, in the dark, I wasn't even sure that I wanted to or that I knew how to. It was physically numbing and emotionally crippling. The only way that I can describe it is that it was like a rubber band being stretched to breaking point. It felt like a dull thud came from somewhere deep within my chest. The sensation reverberated throughout my body. In that moment, my body gave me its most defining message to date—that it was broken, and it had changed. It felt not only as though my heart had changed, but that it had given up. It was encouraging my mind to do the same—to surrender to the pain that was engulfing me. I recognised the feeling instantly, even though I'd never experienced anything close to it before.

That was when I knew I had a choice.

I had to find a way forward or a way out. I was enduring a breakdown as a result of a break-up, which served as the prequel to my eventual *breakthrough*. I didn't want to die, but this version of living was emotionally killing me. In the following months, I chose to move forward—and I'm still choosing that option. I'm travelling, faltering and hoping, putting one foot in front of the other and trying to heal. The final number in the musical Hamilton is "Who lives, Who Dies, Who Tells Your Story?" I'm telling you my story in the hope that my experiences and my words might support, strengthen, and empower you, so that you can edit and rewrite your story. So that you imagine and create a happier ending for yourself; the ending you deserve. Your journey might take you to some emotionally challenging places, but I believe these will be better than the place you're trying to leave behind. As I moved forward, I gradually saw that my worth was not defined by anyone else's ability or lack thereof to see and appreciate it. I know that the same is also true for you. The hardest lessons we learn are the ones that teach us the most. I aim to take you on a journey of self-discovery that will ultimately lead to self-appreciation and self-love, which is greater than anything we can receive from others. Your heart will be stronger and more grateful to you for it.

I offer you my experiences in the hope they become your glue, to restore whichever parts of you that you feel are most in need of repair.

I've always been blindsided by break-ups. Regardless of where, how or when they occurred, the pain has always been overwhelming and as physical as it was emotional. I've gone from standing on cloud nine to being trapped in a frozen lake of self-deprecation, with fresh ice forming in the aftermath, further paralysing me and alienating me from reality. I've lost myself, time and again, as a result of losing another person from my life. Their choice resulted in the latest death-sentence to my self-esteem, and the future I yearned for and thought I saw unfolding. It's like watching your favourite film, the one with the happy-ever-after ending you know by heart, only now, the ending has been rewritten. Your favourite character has died, the wolf has removed its woollen clothes, and you're confronted with the knowledge that nothing was as it seemed, and nothing will ever be the same again.

This might all sound like a dramatic over-reaction to some people, but if you've chosen to read this book, this emotional response may resonate. Ultimately, there's no rule book or blueprint to a break-up, or indeed any right way of reacting to, and recovering from, life-altering news or circumstances beyond your control. What I'm still learning, however, is that the relationship we have with ourselves is the foundation to everything we experience in life. External relationships only survive and sustain us if they're built upon the foundation of us truly knowing and loving the person we are—on our best days and our worst. The intention is to stand tall, proud, and purposeful, both in company and in solitude. Easier said than done, I know.

I've always had an issue with people in a couple being referred to as a 'half', for instance, when someone asks, 'How's your other/better half?' This isn't my opinion because I'm single; however, being single has helped me realise how negative and dehumanising that sentiment is. Of those eight billion people on Earth, if you'd never had contact with any of them during your life, you would still be no more or less of a person than if you spent every waking hour in the company of others. Your existence isn't given value by your interactions or intimacy with others. It isn't negated if you're 'unattached' or living in social isolation, nor is it validated by others. You're never half a person, regardless of your circumstances or relationship status. You're complete, just as you are, for all that you are. No other person can determine, define or be responsible for your level of wholeness. And yet, all the love society encourages us to find, nurture, and invest in is predominantly external. It's rooted within something, anything, outside of ourselves. The relationship we have with ourselves is the most enduring relationship we will ever have. It's the one we enter into from birth, before we have any awareness of others and before we even understand what a relationship is. It's the one connection that will die only when we do.

Recently, an increasing number of love songs have begun to be directed inwards. Miley Cyrus sang, 'I can love me better than you can'; Jess Glynne acknowledged, 'I feel like I've been missin' me', and Demi Lovato pondered, 'I'm an expert at giving love to somebody else, I wonder when I love me is enough.' Before any of these songs were penned, however, Tina Turner asked, 'What's love got to do with it?' With regards to being self-fulfilled and self-reliant, the answer is love has got *everything* to do with it. In its most pure and permanent state, love comes from within. Without meaning to state the obvious, love can only be recognised and achieved externally in our lives when we have it in ourselves, from ourselves. Love may be many things. It may be a many splendid thing. It may make the world go around. It may lift us up where we belong. It may be blind or at least a little colour-blind. It may be just a game, or it may be all we need...whatever love is, it needs to start from within.

I'm obsessed with quotes and positive

affirmations. One that really resonates with me is this: **speak to yourself the way you would to someone you love.**

It got me thinking; if you had to list all the people in your life that you love, how long would it take before you added yourself to that list? How far down would your name feature, if, in fact, it featured at all?

We each know ourselves better than anyone else will ever know us. We spend more time with ourselves than we will with anyone else, and we know the sound of our own voice more instinctively and intimately than that of any other human on the planet. Yet we allow our voice to be drowned out by the views and judgements of others. We allow them to define and break us, whilst we accept loneliness as the companion of our own company in the wake of their absence.

You've been with yourself throughout every living moment you've ever experienced.

You've heard and felt your heart beat repeatedly until you took it for granted, only becoming aware of it during or in the aftermath of exercise, when it beats out of your chest in exhilarated triumph. Or, like I did, in the wake of tragedy, when it silently surrenders to grief.

You have a pair of ears and one tongue. Despite this, we often talk to be heard and hear very little of the messages we receive from within. The more positive they are, the less we take note of them.

You have a voice, but you allow it to be silenced by the opinions of others or the negative monologue from within your mind.

You have a reflection, which is sometimes admired, potentially ignored, and frequently compared and critiqued. Occasionally, it's reduced to a wobbling portrait of pain, regret, and dissatisfaction.

You have eyes that often miss the beauty that's before them, as they search for more, for different, for better. As they look anywhere but inwards for fear of what they may find.

You already have everything within you that you could ever need to survive and thrive. Yet we focus on the aspects and elements of ourselves that we believe to be missing or broken, rather than the potential of all the tools we carry—unused and unappreciated when compared to those of others.

We look at the surface and forget that we're so much more than flesh and self-proclaimed flaws. There's an entire history, present, and future within us, below the surface. It spans a lifetime, but we underestimate it, sell it short, and strive to rewrite it. We become so used to looking at ourselves that we reach a point where we stop seeing ourselves. We look at all the separate pieces without appreciating the whole, unique picture.

If you were to look in the mirror right now, what one thing would you choose to love about yourself?

This won't be an easy question for everyone to answer, but then it isn't meant to be. Often, the harder the question is to ask, the more profound and possibly painful the answer will be.

Some people might struggle to find just one thing; plenty of individuals look upon themselves with love, appreciation, and pride. If this is you, I applaud and admire you. Continue to blow your own trumpet, from every social media platform and to everyone in your contacts. Don't ever hide that light, and don't ever lose your vision or your voice. Self-love is not an ugly trait; it's the absolute opposite.

For many others, however, this is an alien concept. There's no curriculum that teaches us how to look at ourselves with love, respect, pride, and forgiveness. If we learn to do this at all, it's through multiple life lessons in varying degrees of severity. We're led to believe that we'd be committing a crime of vanity if we were to celebrate our existence, our achievements, and our authentic selves. By giving ourselves permission to recognise our beauty and worth and have our moment in the light, we allow that light to permeate the cracks of our imperfections.

If you struggle to look beyond your physical 'flaws' and 'imperfections'; if you've become numb or blind to your worth and potential, please know that you're not alone. You're human, responding to what you see whilst carrying the echoes of everything that has come before it.

Please try to believe me when I tell you:

You are not your insecurities or the secrets you hide. You're the strength that keeps on going and the discretion that protects you.

You are not your unwashed hair or the bags under your eyes. You're a busy person who puts the needs of others above your own self-care or indulgences.

You are not the personification of the perception of others. You're the other side of the story and the magic behind the illusion.

You are not withdrawn or detached. You're the dignity that sits in quiet contemplation, speaking your truth to those who will listen to what is said in the silence.

You are not reserved. Your presence is reserved for those who value the gift of your time.

You and I

You are not every mistake you've ever made. You're the bravery of every attempt you make.

You are not a weight, a measurement, an age or a statistic. You're a complex calculation of every piece of evidence that proves your uniqueness and value.

You are not broken. You're healing. You're breathing. You're trying.

You are not unlovable or hard to love; you just gave your commitment to someone who was unwilling or incapable of matching and returning it. You're not responsible for anyone else's limitations.

There will always be people who will notice and convey the things you're not, rather than all the miraculous things you are. Those who will always see the end result—rather than the journey, the courage or the good intentions it took you to get there. If our hearts and minds healed as quickly as our bones do, there would be no requirement for break-up songs, therapy, self-help books or king-size boxes of tissues and chocolates.

It's all very well to advocate for you to love yourself, but this is the icing on the cake that comes with time, practice, and persistence. We need to bake the cake first, and by that, I mean we need to get to know ourselves and all that there is to understand, respect, and admire, before love can develop and we're able to rise. You'll always know yourself better than anyone else will, even the other human(s) on this earth you're closest to. You are never closer to anyone else than the person who walks within you, who shares your shoes, your skin, your soul, your secrets and your shadow. You are the one person alive who knows every one of your innermost thoughts—including those too raw, unpolished, and destructive to whisper aloud. You are your own secret-keeper, judge, jury and executioner. You're the one person you cannot successfully lie to or evade.

You're the only person who can find, store, and protect your version of happiness. When you do, you must bury it deeply within your identity. Your happiness belongs to you. Other people or groups should only ever be enhancements to your happiness, rather than the custodians of it. Yet this is so rarely the case. We know our potential better than anyone else, but we so often let the expectations of others define us and keep us small. We all have parts of ourselves that are hurting through physical or emotional pain. We carry on, often hoping that no one will notice or judge us for whatever sticking plaster we choose to use to treat the wound. We fail to see the strength that's there, the strength that's silent and stubborn and which refuses to give in. Sometimes, the best way to know ourselves well enough to love ourselves as we deserve to be loved is to step away from the mirror and look within. With unflinching, non-judgemental, and grateful eyes, we need to read our story from the beginning, chapter by poignant chapter, to anticipate a better ending —the one we truly deserve.

We are human—so mistakes, ill-judgement, misplaced trust, and words delivered in uncensored emotion are a given. They undeniably come with the job of being a person. Rather than accepting that these outcomes are par for the course, we carry them as labels. We buckle under their weight and forget how far we've come and how much we've grown when we look ahead at our goals and dreams on the horizon. We're complex and layered.

We are:
- Light and shade
- Hope and despair
- Resilient and fallible
- Forgiving and vengeful
- Laughter and tears
- Perfectly imperfect contradictions

We're all of our ugly truths, but we're never ugly.

We can be beautifully messy, chaotically organised, and bittersweet. Only once we recognise and accept the juxtapositions that arise from being human can we appreciate that this is exactly who we're supposed to be. Unless we've hurt someone on our journey as a human being, we don't need to offer any apologies for being one. Often, the person we owe the biggest apology to is ourselves— for being too quick to meet humanity with destructive negativity, and for our reluctance to forgive ourselves and move on.

A moment to reflect

With this in mind, I would encourage you to take time to think about yourself. Allow unfiltered words to come into your mind. Say them out loud, write them down—whatever you feel most comfortable with. Notice them. Notice how many are complimentary and kind, and how many are self-deprecating or self-destructive. There will likely be a mix of the two, usually weighted towards one extreme or the other. Before you absorb these words, these character traits or character assassinations, consider honestly: how many of them are unbiased and, more importantly, true?

They will all be biased to some degree or other, but are they based on a single event, a snapshot in time or a response to something emotive, rather than a natural, subconscious response, as automatic as breathing? How many have been fed to you by others and which do you truly believe?

Consider all the definitions, labels, and judgements you've placed upon yourself and, once you've decided that they're an honest representation of yourself, take each one in turn and unwrap it, layer by layer. Give it context. Give it a fair hearing. Give it the space to be, before you decide if it's a positive or a negative—a light to bask in or a noose to hang yourself with. Regardless of what you decide and the labels you're left with, remember that they're each a complex piece of the person you are. It's for you to decide whether you want to change them or make peace with them.

Doing this task myself, I'd say that I'm a sensitive person. On the surface, I wouldn't recommend or perceive this trait too favourably, as it can lead you to feel more, absorb more, and think and worry in excess—a sponge permanently saturated by life. However, I've come to realise that being a sensitive person brings empathy and the ability to love more, to appreciate more, and to have deeper feelings. These lead to deeper relationships and more meaningful experiences. This depth of feeling can be devastating if you drown in it, or if you deplete your reserves whilst sustaining others, but life is too short to live at surface level. I've come to realise that the more you're prepared to give of yourself, the more meaningful, rich, and memorable your interactions and experiences will be. Being a sensitive person can carry social stigmas, but it can also bring closeness and strengthen bonds. I'm now learning to manage my thoughts, rather than allowing them to manage me.

Hopefully, once you've taken the time to think of yourself as a whole being, with compartments, layers, and dimensions, you'll have plenty of pieces that make up the full picture of all that you are. Some of these pieces will be visible to the naked eye, whereas some will only be seen through introspection. All your pieces are valid. The challenge comes in recognising, naming, and accepting them with kindness. The challenge comes in seeing the bigger picture of why you became this version of yourself, and how to use those pieces as your armour rather than a stick to beat yourself with. They are each a part of your story and identity, and you shouldn't be ashamed of them.

The most crucial part of this process is to be

sure that every internal word you hear is yours and not something fed to you by others—as, often, external voices speak the loudest. Just to clarify, you're not expected to like every part of yourself or to view every trait glowingly; each imperfection is simply part of being a human being. You're a work in progress, and every experience takes you further along your journey. We all rise, fall and adapt—that's part of evolution and life as a human. By recognising the parts of ourselves we might see less favourably, we get to make a choice; to either accept them, challenge them or change them (or any of the circumstances within our lives that enable them). Make that decision for yourself, but remember that any change you make is just as much a work in progress as you are.

Once you've begun the journey of recognising and accepting who you are and all that you are, it's important to remember that the process of learning to love ourselves is exactly that: a lesson that begins in our earliest years that we never fully complete. It's a purposeful, daily pursuit that requires love and perseverance. It will be easier to do it on some days than others, and that's okay. Use the good days to strengthen you for the more challenging ones. Use the memories and people you've collected along the way to support you. Like positive pebbles, they can become the foundation to your self-acceptance and appreciation, and the basis of the life you truly want to live.

You are life-giving, life-sustaining, and life-enhancing, but you're not a tree. You have the capacity to grow, withstand and thrive, but you also have the opportunity to branch out in whichever direction serves you best. You can take root in the environment that strengthens you most naturally, for as long as that may be. If your circumstances or environment become hostile rather than healthy, give yourself the permission to move, to improve, and to live with different views and opportunities. Don't settle where you feel you've been planted. Don't settle for any aspect of your life that doesn't reflect or respect who you are. Follow your dreams and potential, and all that you're capable of being.

Mirror, mirror

Mirror, mirror, on the wall,
who will catch me when I fall?

Take a look at me
and tell me what you see.
Tell me honestly.
I don't need a sycophant.
I'm not being petulant.
I'm someone who tries too hard,
someone scared, someone scarred.
Life has thrown a curveball,
it's had me up against a wall,
until I don't recognise the me I see,
but is that such a travesty?
I can change, I can grow;
stand up, move on, let it go.
Learn from all that was said and done,
accept the me I have become.
We're not so different, you and me,
we share the same reality.
I will stumble, I will soar.
I won't apologise anymore.
I see white hairs where there were none.
Does this mean my youth has gone?
You show me weight, lost and gained;
I show you a heart in pain.
You show me eyes, raw and red;

should I share with you the thoughts in my head?
I am all you will ever see,
where there is you, there I will be.
I won't always get it right,
but I'll walk through darkness to the light.
Often out of sight, but always real,
you wear the scars of all I feel.
I reach a hand out to you,
the parting gift I always do.

Mirror, mirror, on the wall,
I will catch me if I fall.

Do you know who you are? Do you know what has happened to you?

We should perhaps consider these questions as two different branches stemming from the same tree. The answer is rooted in our brain development, and how it enables us to process what is happening to and around us, the experiences we've had, the events we've lived through and the lessons we've learned. It controls how we make sense of each experience—in the moment, in the mirror, and in retrospect. As we reflect upon our reflection, the mirror has the potential to present us with half-truths, half the story, and blatant lies. We contemplate the lines age habitually carves into the skin we secretly seek to shed. We view the core standing before the mirage of the rounded apple, which retreats in shame. We consider the chameleon fighting against nature to keep its emotions concealed in the cold light of day. Maybe these questions should really be considered the other way around. By first understanding, processing, and accepting what has happened to us, we can begin to form a nurturing relationship with the person who's been created as a result. The answers to these questions are likely to be as changeable and as inconsistent as we are.

Around week six of a pregnancy, the process of growing and developing a life-sustaining brain begins. This continues throughout pregnancy and during the next two-and-a-half decades of our lives. During these ensuing twenty-five years (approximately 9,125 days), a neurotypical brain will navigate the intricacies and complexities of the following survival skills:

- Early language and communication
- Movement
- Forming and sustaining relationships
- Self-care
- Decision making and self-advocacy
- Making choices and understanding consequences

- Morality and fairness

All of these developmental milestones are interlaced with the responsibilities of meeting societal expectations, pressures, and demands. If you think about it, from the moment we're born, we're exposed to experiences that require us to react and adapt in order to survive. Our neurological development, and all that has played a part in moulding it, determines our ability to respond to challenges and choices. What that response may look like, what it may demand of us, and what its implications may be on the rest of our lives, cannot be predicted. Each decision our brain makes causes a ripple effect, which can resonate for seconds, days, decades—or, potentially, an entire lifetime.

In week six or seven of gestation, the brain separates into three parts: the front brain, the midbrain, and the hindbrain. These will eventually develop into the complex parts of the brain responsible for governing our survival responses, our emotional responses, and our thinking and reasoning skills. At this point, the brain will expand and develop at a rate of 250,000 neurons per minute for the next twenty-one weeks. At birth, a baby is already equipped with almost all of the brain cells or neurons that it will ever have throughout its life—approximately eighty-six billion.

The survival brain, scientifically referred to as the brain stem and cerebellum, is located within the hindbrain. As the name suggests, it's responsible for ensuring our survival from dangers from one day to the next, both within and outside of ourselves. This is the part of the brain that assessed danger from predators in primitive times. It's also the part that babies are most dependent upon within the womb, and during their earliest, most developmentally-significant years. It's effectively your control centre, which can either shut down your body in the face of danger—physically and emotionally paralysing you with fear—or send you running for the hills as fast as your lungs and legs will allow. As a third option, your adrenal glands release a rush of the stress-regulating hormone cortisol. This floods your body in response to perceived stress and danger, directing messages like an alarm system throughout your body, providing the required energy to instinctively fight for your survival. Our fight-flight-freeze response, directed by our 'survival brain', is a commonly used and recognised term to represent our reaction to stress. Mental Health First Aid England also acknowledges, in its first-aider training programme, a fourth 'F': flatulence. This reaction sees your body try to empty itself with immediacy and urgency. It acts as a means of asserting control over a hostile situation in which it feels held captive. Ridding itself of everything it feels is a toxin or an unnecessary weight in the body increases its flight response. As someone who lives with irritable bowel syndrome, this fourth F is as real as it is inconvenient. That which originates in the mind doesn't always stay there and the gut is referred to as our second brain for good reason.

Whilst this part of the brain deals with how we recognise danger, the midbrain is concerned with processing and regulating our emotional responses to what we encounter and socially engage with. It's the part of our brain that provides the multi-dimensional sensory input to our experiences. It adds the visual and auditory landscape (i.e. the texture, taste and the scent) to each memory we make. It's also where memories are stored for future reference and safe-keeping. The survival and emotional parts of our brain are interconnected and reliant upon one another to recognise and interpret situations, and to determine the level of emotional response they require— from joy to fear, and everything in-between.

The largest part of the brain, and the last to be fully developed, is the forebrain. This is comprised of the cerebrum, cerebral cortex, and thalamus. The forebrain provides us with the ability to learn, to retain and recall information, to solve problems, to understand concepts and ideas, and to think empathetically. Whilst our survival brain sees a a problem, and our emotional brain works out how we feel about the situation and gauges the level of threat, our thinking brain allows us to understand the situation and generate an appropriate response. Whether you act first and think later or think before you react is determined by the part of your brain that kicks in first. This decides how rational, reactive or emotional a person you are in any given moment.

Our survival brain forms first, being the most primitive and alert element. The thinking and rational brain is the largest and takes longer to develop. It's comparable to a house requiring the foundations to be laid before the structure can be erected. How solid and stable this structure is for the lifetime we inhabit it depends upon how consistent and positive our experiences are.

Our lives can be affected by the extent to which we find ourselves living in survival mode to navigate and remain in control of our environment and circumstances. For example, if we lived in a constant state of high-alert, due to the presence of a perceived or tangible threat, we would not be able to enjoy successful, deep, and sustaining relationships, nor a high level of emotional wellbeing or social involvement. We wouldn't develop the capabilities to personally and professionally thrive; we'd merely be surviving. Our foundations are laid in the womb and, once we enter the world, we're exposed to experiences that will either strengthen or weaken them. The more stress we experience, the more we must fight to adapt and survive, and the greater the consequences for the rest of our future fulfilment.

As humans, little in our lives is certain. There's a limit to what we can predict or control. We can't always know how much stress we'll encounter or the form that stress will take. The more stress we experience, however, the more resilient and reactive our brains strive to be. In turn, this brings a greater impact on our overall wellbeing, and ultimately, the quality and longevity of our lives.

We may experience three types of stress during our lives, either in isolation to or in conjunction with each other:

Acute stress is something I have no doubt

everyone has experienced. Our body goes into a sudden state of shock, based on an immediate and unforeseen situation—with potentially life-threatening, dangerous or unpleasant repercussions. Acute stress can be triggered by events such as narrowly avoiding a road accident or an attack, sleeping through your alarm and dealing with being late for something, or assisting with, witnessing, or experiencing a medical emergency. Such incidents are usually isolated and infrequent, but each one is stored in our memory banks and can affect and determine how we respond to future levels and forms of threat.

Chronic stress is typically endured over a sustained period of time. Whilst the threat isn't immediate, its effect is no less damaging. With each potentially back-breaking straw, placed precariously on top of others, the structure of your life risks eventual collapse – with mental, physical or emotional consequences. Dreading going to work every day, living in an unhappy or unhealthy relationship or home environment, or coping with a long-term medical condition, can all be a catalyst for chronic stress. Such situations see us rely on our innate survival instinct, which increases the level of cortisol in our bodies.

Finally, there is **traumatic stress**. This

typically creates a sense of helplessness or sustained fear, due to a lack of control over the situation or its outcome. Examples of traumatic stress include living through a war, homelessness, a physical assault, extreme weather or a natural disaster. An event that causes traumatic stress, or a secondary response of post-traumatic stress disorder (PTSD), usually involves the roles of a perpetrator and survivor. Experiencing this kind of stress pre-adulthood, during our most formative and fragile stages of development, is known as an ACE (Adverse Childhood Experience). The more ACEs we experience, or the greater the severity of an ACE, the more lasting and detrimental the effects can be throughout the remainder of our lives. More so if we're not adequately equipped or supported enough to understand what we've been through and how to begin the healing process.

An ACE is a recognised term to describe adverse childhood experiences that could have a detrimental impact on an individual's physical development and mental health. This vulnerability could affect their future opportunities and life expectancy. According to Gloucestershire Healthy Living and Learning, 48% of adults in England have experienced at least one ACE. If this rises to six ACEs before the age of eighteen, their life expectancy could be reduced by twenty years.

An ACE was initially defined under three categories of trauma: physical, emotional or sexual abuse; physical or emotional neglect; or negative family circumstances. The latter may include domestic violence, parental separation and divorce, parental imprisonment, mental illness or substance abuse.

More recently, further life experiences were added to this broad definition. An ACE is now categorised as:
- being bullied or experiencing discrimination
- being a witness to the bullying or abuse of a sibling
- seeing someone threatened or attacked with a gun or knife
- living in an unsafe neighbourhood or having to flee your home or country due to danger
- experiencing a consistently inconsistent home life, due to repeatedly moving home or school
- the loss of a close family member
- being taken into or moving through foster care
- experiencing extreme illness or injury that either affects them personally or a close family member

These definitions may seem extreme, but

our worldview is changing on a daily basis. We're increasingly digesting a more emotionally-challenging diet, which has the potential to poison us from the outside in if we cannot protect ourselves from the inside out. Recent research by ITV highlighted a 40% decline in the mental health of school-aged children across England since 2019. It showed that they're increasingly worried about, and aware of, whether their families have enough money to provide life's necessities. They're worried about wars in other countries and how they could affect them, as well as the threat posed by climate change. These are detrimentally heavy loads to be carried by any human, particularly ones so small and emotionally unequipped, with so little life experience behind them. They have very little to steady and protect them against the onslaught of events that lie beyond their control.

As we've already discussed, the reactive part of our brain that's responsible for maintaining our survival is the most primitive, and the first to develop. It's our go-to response in stressful, dangerous situations and, just like any other muscle in the body, the more we use it, the stronger its reflexes and responses become. Put another way, the more traumas we encounter in our life, the quicker we become to react, physically or emotionally, in order to keep ourselves safe. As a result, however, we become less able to engage with life on a level of deep joy, self-love, and appreciation—because this is not our first instinct. In such a scenario, that part of our brain doesn't speak the loudest; it feels less familiar to us and it doesn't offer any physical protection or safety.

If this is the case for you, know that you're reacting in the way that comes most naturally. This may have become your default, your emotional crutch or your practical safety blanket. If you have one significant adverse experience behind you or multiple experiences that have accumulated in your initial chapters, it may feel as though they've set the scene and the tone of your ensuing story. But they do not define your character, and they're not your fault. They do not decide what your future chapters will hold; they're not a group of malevolent authors with pens poised over the remaining blank pages of your life story. Whether you've experienced adversity in childhood, or whether such experiences come to you later in life, (which I am referring to as adverse life experiences or ALEs), your responses will be shaped by the decisions your brain makes. It might offer you an escape route, e.g. fighting back, fleeing the situation, residing in denial or turning to others for comfort and protection. Remember: our brains continue to develop, mature, and adapt until we're approximately twenty-five-years-old. The strength and success of our responses to traumas and adversity usually depends on how many years we've lived and the quality of the life that has been lived during that time. Your body can equip you with all you need to survive, despite the hostility of the environment it might find itself in. That's the miraculous beauty and the unique strength of your body. I think we all need to face and free ourselves from our adverse life experiences with patience and compassion—one step and one day at a time. You're not what has happened to you, nor are you a product of what you've lived through. You are a survivor of all that has come before.

Throughout the pages of this book, I make the point that we are each made of gold. I feel so strongly about this that I've embedded it within the title.

Our gold is our mental strength, our emotional resilience, and our individual drive to get up and move forward.

It's our ability to fly, to flourish, and to feel.

It's our determination to find freedom on a daily basis, and to heal from the inside out, from whatever may have burned, broken or scarred us.

It's the gift of being able to inspire others to heal, love, and live again.

What we have been through refers to the experiences we've had and the emotions we felt as a result. Who we are is the unique and precious gold that lies beneath the layers we wear to protect ourselves. It's the kindness, love, and hope that sit quietly, yet resolutely, within us all. It's what creates the person we are; and when we're stripped back and laid bare, what life cannot touch or taint.

Rather than make an inspiring analogy between the precious elements of our character and a precious natural element, I'll explain the science behind my words. Every one of us holds a tiny yet significant amount of gold within us. In a human body weighing 70kg, this equates to 0.2 milligrams. Most of the body's gold is found within the brain, joints, blood, and heart, and it carries many recognised health benefits. Given that blood is transferred around the body from the heart, this suggests to me an unscientifically proven yet tenable link to the adage 'a heart of gold'.

Earlier this year, I went for a walk with my dad. We noticed fungi growing on a felled branch, and he said something far more profound than I was expecting for a Sunday afternoon: life grows on death. This made me think of many things. The way we can miss the gift of connection and all that our senses present us with when we're not fully present in the moment. It reminded me that a negative situation can produce and sustain a positive outcome. Light can penetrate darkness, like the sun's rays breaking through the clouds.

I know of people whose ACEs or ALEs have:
- led them to God
- led them to the career they were born to do
- led them to the family they were destined to have
- led them to a version of happiness or a level of love they never thought they would experience
- led them to heal and fulfil their potential, and enable a better relationship with themselves

If you've lived through any form of adversity or you're currently navigating your way through pain, I hope that you're able to recognise the undeniable worth within yourself that sits quietly, waiting to be called upon to strengthen you.

Do you know what has happened to you? Have you taken the time to consider, to address, and to heal from the experiences you've had in your life up to this point? Have you considered how adverse or favourable those experiences were, and what impact they had? Have you taken a moment to look back on all that has happened and which has led to the decisions you make today?

Do you know what you've lived through? Do you know what you've survived? Do you know what or who has strengthened you, tested you or empowered you? Do you know the significance of each event? Do you see them in isolation, or do you see them as conjoining pieces of a bigger picture?

If you were to put 100 people in a room together, it's guaranteed that each one of them would be utterly unique. Even if their age, upbringing, life experiences, and opportunities were (impossibly) identical, it's still highly probable that their individual neurological reactions to the lives they've lived would be different. However similar our experiences are, it's our natural tendencies to instinctively lean towards surviving, emotionally experiencing the world or internally rationalising our experiences that set us apart. That's the beauty of being human. We all bring something completely unique to the table, whatever that table looks like. The more adverse your life experiences are, whether in childhood or beyond, the greater their effect on the quality of your life. If you're constantly living in a state of high alert, awaiting the next danger or struggle to arrive, it will be a battle to live in the moment or be appreciative of anyone or anything else. If you've got a catalogue of ACEs or ALEs behind you that you haven't made peace with, you won't be completely free to explore or experience who it is that you could be, who you want be, or who you're capable of being.

You're a perfectly imperfect human. You're made up of a unique blend of chemicals, survival instincts, emotional responses, and thought processes—all contained within a body that's uniquely yours and which requires no apologies. You've survived 100% of your worst days; you're more than an accumulation of all that's ever happened to you. You're a survivor of the experiences that scarred but which didn't define you. You're surviving and living and defining yourself on your own terms, and that's enough. If you're struggling to process or make peace with any of the life experiences you've lived through or you need help and support to manage your emotional reactions to them, there are organisations listed at the end of this book that may be able to provide the support strategies, resources, and opportunities to aid your emotional recovery.

Breathe

*When did you last breathe
and notice every breath?
Did you take the time to realise
each one was the difference between life and death?*

*Have you ever really listened to your heart
with silence instrumental to each beat?
Did you stop to allow your toes to explore
the foundations that lay at their feet?*

*Have you stopped to listen to
the child who is still inside?
Who is serving time for adulthood's crimes
yet despite it all, they have not died.*

*They are yearning for you to chase
bubbles as much as dreams
and remember that reality
can be so much more than all it seems.*

*Do you ever feel the stirrings
as they gently take your hand
and promise you adventures
in a long-forgotten land?*

On the surface it's not so different

from the one you have come to know.
You just have to look deep within,
believe in yourself and let go.

When did you last have ice cream for breakfast,
plant a seed to watch it grow,
become a mermaid with a tail of sand,
or dare to mix the colours of the play dough?

Have you made a wish lately
on a dandelion or a shooting star?
Or laid in the grass and looked to the sky
and realised how small you truly are?

Have you found animals in the clouds
and been enchanted by the sun,
as it bleeds the memories of a day
that started with such promise, but which now,
is almost done?

So, give that child back their voice
and listen as they remind you
to take a breath in this moment
and simply enjoy, with gratitude, the view.

A counsellor told me years ago that to live in the past brings about depression, and to live in the future leads to a state of anxiety. The past cannot be physically changed, revisited or rewritten. Yet we replay it repeatedly like a torturous film marathon, where the cinema is our mind, and all escape routes are blocked by 'what ifs' and pain. The future is often out of sight and outside of our control. Still, we try and outrun and outsmart it, in an attempt to be forewarned and forearmed; to be a formidable opponent to our anxieties. With one eye permanently cast behind us on a path already travelled, we're bound to fall over past recriminations, which encourage old wounds to resurface and bleed—fatally, if we allow them. If our other eye is looking to the horizon, we'll miss the path beneath us, which may be paved with gold or peppered with sinkholes to avoid. Life happens in the present. Whatever has come before is a memory. Whatever is yet to come isn't promised or predictable.

For more than half my lifetime, I've carried a suitcase full of emotional scars from place to place. I've unpacked it regularly and allowed it to taint my today and tarnish my tomorrow. I've lived with the regrets of missed opportunities, the pain of rejection, the devastation of decisions made, and the impact of words both thought and spoken. The past has caused elements of my future to slip through my fingers...shards of broken dreams and shattered self-esteem. It's taken me a lifetime to realise that the present is all there is, and it passes in a heartbeat as we breathe one breath after another.

I've heard it said that whilst we, as adults, teach children all about life, it's children, when given the chance, who teach us what life is all about. I'm not sure at what point childhood ends and life as we know it, with all its constraints, expectations, rules, and requirements, takes over. It seems increasingly apparent to me that there's an endpoint to childhood and the freedom it brings. Maybe it's when we step over puddles, rather than jumping into them with wild abandon. Maybe it's when we stop singing and dancing as if our lives depended on it and we instead reserve such an act for the shower, the car, the kitchen or some other solitary space. Perhaps it's when we look at our reflections with criticism, rather than with appreciation and curiosity. Possibly, it's when time shifts from an abstract, meaningless concept, to the invisible hands that govern our waking moments. We live in a world that increasingly expects and encourages us to be busy. To continually be doing and achieving, with the focus on the end result, rather than the process of simply 'being'. Don't get me wrong, I understand that we all have roles to play in life and contributions to make, and that we must show up in order to do them. We have to grow, learn, flourish, and adapt. We need to accept the responsibility that comes with being alive, as we meet the needs and expectations of ourselves and others. To be clear, I'm not advocating for a dereliction of adult duties as we each personify Peter Pan. But I have noticed that we've become resolute in our pursuit of shaping children, at an increasingly early age, to be ready for our world —rather than preparing our world to be fit and ready for our children.

We seem to be on an incessant mission to prepare our children to reach our milestones, to our timescales, at a perilously young and tender age. To be ready for a formal way of learning, for being tested and categorised, and to have developed specific knowledge and a predetermined skill set before they've even developed a sense of self. To fit into a box, when their natural instincts are screaming to be heard and seen as an individual, and when they most need support to spread their fragile, emerging wings. We expect so much of children —often seeing them as little humans whose sole purpose is to grow into bigger humans, rather than acknowledging and celebrating the fact that their only job is to be an authentic and individual child. Childhood is such a short season. By reducing the length and quality of that precious period, we're determining the shape and success of every season that follows.

My point is that children are magical. They believe in magic, and they create magic within the everyday things adults become immune and indifferent to. They make wishes upon dandelions, which become magical wands to transform others into a unicorn, which can fly to the moon and splash in the oceans, with mermaids and piranha fish. They can be chased by a megalodon, pausing only to fight giant gingerbread people, who live in jewel-encrusted sandcastles that are guarded by fairies and superheroes. It all sounds highly improbable, fanciful, and time-consuming, but imagine the possibilities and the simple joy of seeing something for all it could be, rather than everything we're told it is. I work with young children who take you by the hand every day and drag you at full speed through endless adventures in imagined realities; who continually describe spontaneous missions and journeys of discovery. It's exhausting, but I feel endlessly grateful for their trust, vulnerability, and honesty. I feel privileged that they force me from my grown-up world of anxieties, inadequacies, and responsibilities and into their world of living for and in the moment, which they accept exactly as it is. Last year, at home time, one of my children greeted his parent with, 'This is the best day of my life.' Those eight words were immensely weighted, and they carried such authentic happiness and gratitude. His genuine emotions came straight from his heart, resting on his flushed and sincere face. Children don't overthink or over-analyse. They speak with (often brutal) honesty, and if they say something, it's likely because they truly mean, feel, and believe it. That outpouring of happiness was an unfiltered window to his heart and mind in that moment.

When was the last time your inner child uttered those words?

As adults, irrespective of our circumstances, opportunities for happiness seem to come with conditions. Such as, you can enjoy the moment, but keep an eye on the time for your parking. Don't forget to take the dog for a walk, respond to that email or start dinner. Joy seems to come hand in hand with a pocket watch. We may not be children anymore and we may not all have children in our lives, but we all have a child within us. When given the opportunity, they will pull at our hand, turn a moment from the mundane to the magical, and they'll show us how to view the world with awe and wonder—however briefly. Those moments are a gift.

You don't have to be a child to have a childlike appreciation or to see the possibilities or beauty in a situation. Awe and wonder doesn't have to come with an expiry date. You just have to be present in the moment and embrace it for all it is. See how big and meaningful the smallest of things can be. Be present and mindful, rather than being preoccupied and 'mind-full'. Consider the magic of a murmuration, the significance of a sunset, and the joy of shared laughter. If we open our eyes to all that there is to see and open our hearts to all that there is to feel, we can become richer, wiser, and better as a result. By being aware of, and appreciating the moment, our glass can be both repaired and replenished.

Going for a walk during the Coronavirus lockdowns was a surreal experience. The natural world responded to the enforced change of pace and human senses became heightened to the stillness, the brightness, and the quietness that emerged. Nature seemed to flourish as humans retreated. If you were present enough, you became part of it. Lockdowns felt like either a lifetime or a life sentence at the time, but now that time has, on the most part, become an uncertain memory.

Back then, we were forced to slow down. Now that life has returned to full-speed, full-volume, and full-intensity, we must force ourselves to once again stop, notice, and appreciate. We can never predict which breath will be our last. We can never anticipate which moments will become significant. We never know how resilient we can be or how much we value something or love someone until something forces us to find this out.

Perhaps controversially, I think we either live life in the moment or we live life through a lens; we can't do the two simultaneously. In May 2023, I saw an online video as part of a news item that detailed an explosion in Milan. It was thought to have been caused by a truck containing oxygen cylinders. Plumes of smoke engulfed the skyline, sirens punctuated the silence, and carnage and confusion were evident on peoples' faces and in their voices. What I noticed, which was more striking and perhaps more shocking than the scene unfolding, was the fact that everyone in the vicinity was filming it all on their phones—no doubt to share with the world via social media. We're all journalists now, sharing news as it breaks before the news channels arrive. I couldn't help but wonder, if Armageddon played out around us, like a live action horror movie with no potential for a sequel, would we run for our lives? Would we embrace or attempt to rescue our loved ones or would we instead reach for our phones to record it all, for eyes that would never witness it? It seems as though we're increasingly forced to ask ourselves: if it wasn't caught on camera, did it even happen? And how much did it matter?

From experience, don't let the voice of your children, your inner child or those you love become background noise. Notice them, be present amongst them, enjoy and embrace them. Don't ignore the rainbow whilst searching for the pot of gold, whilst shielding your eyes from the sun or dodging the puddles. Appreciate the present for the gift it is, rather than wistfully thinking of it as the present you will never get to reopen. Make memories you'll remember rather than excuses you'll regret. If you can dream it, chase it. Don't be the one who stands in your way.

Breathe to steady yourself. Breathe to calm your mind. Breathe to restart your heart. Breathe to survive, but more than that, breathe to live and remind yourself that you're alive. Breathe to give yourself the strength to survive the storm. Breathe purposefully, with every step you take and each decision you make. Breathe life into each moment. Remember that, in order for a moment to take your breath away, you need to be present in that moment and breathe through all that you experience.

Acts of kindness for your inner child:

Start small and take yourself on a solo sensory walk. Notice everything that a busy life of multi-tasking causes you to miss.

Hear the birdsong, the human interaction or the sound of silence so often lost in the noise.

Smell the scents in your surroundings, e.g. wood burning, a mowed lawn or foliage in bloom.

Feel the shoes encasing your feet with each step, the sensation of drizzle on your skin or the rhythm of your heart beating.

If relevant, taste the salt in the sea air. See not only the objects you pass, but their colours, their shape, their brightness, and their place within the landscape.

Notice the clouds and the shapes they make. Spot faces within the bark of a tree, or the wildlife existing above, beneath, and beside you.

Capture each moment in your mind's eye and your heart. Store it in your memory bank, rather than relying upon a memory stick to prove that you lived through and captured the moment.

Allow your body to feel it all. Your life experiences should be as three-dimensional as you are. They can be the difference between living and existing.

Do you know what has happened to you?

Time wears a white coat

Time.
That greatest invisible magician
that sits idly on our hands,
with no sign of contrition
for its inconsistency of pace,
as it flies in the face of fun
whilst trickling through our fingers as we trace
the sands of time,
along the finite path we tread,
with a blend of optimism and dread,
navigating our way through
the tedious and the sublime
of this poisoned challis we have all been given;
this gift of time.

We are told to spend it wisely,
as it doesn't come with a refund or a guarantee.
It holds its cards close to its chest
as it takes us from abundance to poverty.
We believe there will always be more,
like the gift that keeps on giving.
We make withdrawals,
time after time,
in the pursuit of thriving, surviving and living.
The material is immaterial,
as beg, borrow or steal,
time can neither be bought nor sold,

yet it is priceless in its ability to heal.
There is no instant gratification.
The road to recovery often goes via Hell.
Yet we are told to hang on in there and ride it out
and have faith in the truth that time will tell.
We are told to have patience,
yet time waits for no man.
Take a breath and breathe through the pain
and ignore the irony, if you can.

Time.

That fluctuating friend or foe,
either on our side or against us,
from one moment to the next.
We can only be certain of its ebb and flow.
It offers us its hands
and the allure of a better version of itself,
leading us through the darkness,
to a greater strength, better health and a deeper sense of self.
We grow through what we go through
and emerge on the other side.
Time is our constant companion,
as our hopes and fears collide.

If you could have access to all the money in the world or the guarantee of all the time in the world, which would you choose?

You could surpass the fortune of Elon Musk but you would be as limited as the rest of us with the time you have to spend that wealth. Your material wealth is immaterial when it comes to negotiating the time you have to exist, to live, and to leave a legacy. Both time and money can be sources of immense happiness, security, and opportunities. In reality, however, whilst they promise power and pleasure, their impermanence is the bitter aftertaste of the poisoned apple. All the money and 'stuff' in the world would be of little comfort or relevance if our health was to deteriorate, if our relationships crumbled or our hearts were broken. Our worldly goods would be nothing more than chocolate teapots if we were to navigate our way through the emotional and physical pain of human fallibility and loss.

When faced with life's most brutal and raw realities—including our own mortality—we'd all desperately try to buy ourselves more time. More time on Earth, more time to fight for a cure or a victory. More time to save or savour a relationship or more time to appreciate a person or a moment. We yearn for more time to achieve something, to be someone, to go somewhere. We beg for more time to make a mark, to matter, to make memories; to do it all again and to do it better. We ache to say the things we've never said and do the things we've never done. In our relationship and power-struggle with time, procrastination is our kryptonite. Time will always have the upper hand.

We're reminded to spend time wisely, like any investment. We're told to make it for ourselves as a therapeutic escape. We're encouraged to donate it selflessly as a random act of kindness. We're implored to never waste it in futility or take it for granted. When we treat time with impatience, as something to idle away, endure or pass in boredom—like the trailer or warm-up act to the main event—we miss the point. Time passes quickly when we're enjoying ourselves and it stretches to an eternity when we're idle; both situations can leave us frustrated and resentful of its pace. Time comes and goes, with no obligation to meet our expectations. It has no interest in our emotional reactions to, or investment in, the moment it presents. It has no ability to lengthen, pause, repeat or rewind itself for our convenience or benefit. Time is impartial to our situations and indifferent to our responses to it. It is what it is, and it's up to us to recognise and appreciate it for all that it fleetingly offers us before it's gone forever.

Time wears a white coat

Time passes, regardless of how we utilise it or how meaningful we make it. If we're only passive spectators of it, we cannot expect to actively benefit from it.

They say time is up there with the great and elite healers of pain, wrongs, and injustices. But expecting the passing minutes, hours, and months to cure our heartbreak or mental anguish is like turning up to a hospital waiting room one day and never checking in at reception. Without acknowledgement of the situation, action, and treatment, you will effectively be sitting and bleeding out as you wait for time to do its thing. Time heals only when it's given the necessary tools and permission. Sitting in idle anticipation of emotional recovery will see time pass like planes at an airport. However, unless you board the plane, your view, destination, and experiences will never change.

Time is like two contrasting sides of the same coin. It can be both a numbing anaesthetic and a painful recovery. If we're passive in the anaesthetic stage, we can only heal successfully if we're active in the recovery stage. Healing demands that we're present, reflective, and receptive to every emotional reaction we encounter. We must be aware of our environment—the metaphorical cliff edges, the idyllic sandy shores, and everything in-between—whilst keeping in mind the emotional place we ultimately want to reach.

However, healing isn't a destination. There isn't an end point at which you'll arrive one day. No commemorative selfie by a welcome sign or setting down of roots for the remainder of your days. It isn't a picture-perfect beauty spot, recognisable by a landmark or distance travelled. No one can navigate it for you. Others cannot describe it to you. They can't judge or critique your version of it or decide an acceptable timeframe that your journey will take. You travel alone. You alone bear the weight of the pain and emotions you're carrying, which will inconsistently alter, minute by minute. You arrive alone, in a place where you eventually feel comfortable enough to recognise and share the emotional souvenirs you'll have accumulated along the way.

I believe that life does come with a manual, but it's written in invisible ink. Only by experiencing something are you able to reveal and read the pearls of wisdom, insights, and survivors' tips that will aid your healing and see you through to the next chapter. That ink fades over time. When you live through a similar experience, you must reveal the writing all over again. Once you've endured a soul-destroying experience, you'll be armed with emotions and tools that will serve as the blueprint to your recovery. The chapter entitled 'sadness', however, will read differently to every other that follows it with a similar theme.

It's important to acknowledge that to heal from something isn't ever to 'get over it'. That sentiment is insensitive, unrealistic, and unhelpful. Healing is to get *through* something, to learn to live with it, and to, eventually, become stronger because of and despite it. To describe healing as a journey is more than a metaphor or a hollow cliché. It's just as transformative, purposeful, and unpredictable as any physical journey a human can make. Everyone who approaches the act of healing wants a happy ending, but the preluding pain makes the beginning messy and chaotic. It's a journey that needs to be planned for, which could be both beautiful and brutal at any given moment. It's also as life-sustaining as breathing. If we don't plan for and partake in that journey in the aftermath of pain, that pain will paralyse us from the inside out. It will have won.

Along the way, and in no particular order, we will pass through many landmarks and locations, as we journey from our lowest ebb to higher states. There will be signs for:

- shock
- denial
- anger
- devastation
- confusion
- vengeance
- pain
- acceptance
- numbness
- helplessness
- self-deprecation
- self-sabotage
- optimism
- reflection

We may pass through one state fleetingly, with barely a flicker of an emotional response or sense of belonging. The next may feel so right in the moment that we're enticed to stay for an eternity. We may be briefly *confused* by the turn of events and the way circumstances are unfolding yet dwell in *devastation* for so long that we take root and become firmly implanted in that land. This state may seem to answer all our questions and provide an outlet to our *pain*, which is the river that runs through each land we inhabit. *Vengeance* is like one of those reversible plush toys, with a grumpy expression concealed underneath a soft, smiling outer skin. The slightest word or deed may flip you inside out, until you don't recognise the reflection in front of you or the feelings within you.

Acceptance is a state with a smaller area of *numbness* residing within it; usually, the two claim you as a resident simultaneously. *Denial* often leads you to encounter *vengeance*, once you've outstayed your welcome and others have tried to guide you along a different, healthier path, more rooted in reality.

Whichever emotional states you pass through, dwell in, explore, reject or personify—and for however long—your road to healing will look different to everyone else's. That's more than okay. Others can be there to support you, guide you, and keep you company along the way, facilitating your progress with love. They will stay for varying durations, serve many purposes, and help to navigate the very worst and loneliest of places...if you let them. Ultimately, the journey is yours alone. You're in control of every aspect of it, despite the fact that, along the way, you will likely feel less in control than at any other point in your life. You alone hear the internal war within yourself. You're the only one who will ever experience the silent sensation of your heart breaking. This is your hell, which paves the way to your healing. But whilst you're the only one who will experience your journey, your healing can be determined by the people you spend time with along the way. They can, if you let them, be the difference between wandering, lost and afraid and finding your way home again—stronger, and more hopeful. Where there is a choice, the view always looks brighter and more manageable with someone by your side. Forrest Gump may have run a one-man race, but he was never short of spectators and the support and solidarity he needed to succeed.

You must heal with intent, which involves several things. It involves awareness of the situation you're in. The process of naming it and the emotional places it takes you to. You need the desire to face all the raw, unimaginably hard, and seemingly impossible moments. You must have the intention to collect and acknowledge these moments and their impact, before processing and disempowering them. You must take a breath and say aloud what you're going through, what has happened to you, and how you're feeling as a result. You must acknowledge the pain and your emotional scars. To name all the things you feel before you can overcome their effects. It doesn't have to be public, eloquent or well-thought out—and, honestly, it shouldn't be any of those things. It will likely involve you sat in a heap, tears staining your cheeks as gasps of breath punctuate your cries, whilst your wounded pride or heart shatters the silence through the narration of your pain. Perhaps numbness will replace your tears. Maybe you'll find yourself feeling more like a pumpkin post-Halloween, i.e. hollow, bruised, scarred and violated, than you ever thought it was possible to feel, as you whisper your story into the darkness.

I cannot stress this enough: when you look and feel your most broken and vulnerable, this is when you need help to heal.

Please know that this is never a display or admission of weakness, but rather evidence of your realisation that you can and should fight to live alongside, through, and past your pain. It's the proof of your strength.

I don't always believe in coincidences, but sometimes, events intervene that guide you to exactly where you need to be. Metaphorical doors and windows of opportunity open. A person may come into your life at the most opportune moment, as if their character was purposely written into your story. A chance conversation could change your life.

It was whilst I was sat in my most pumpkin-like state on my kitchen floor in 2015 that something made me drag myself up off my knees and go to that one drawer that everyone seems to have. You know the one...the drawer full of random items that you cannot possibly part with (because, in truth, you have no earthly idea what they are, where they came from, or when you might actually need them). I found a booklet detailing services in my local area that was somehow still in date, and I opened it as if I knew what I was looking for. The truth was I didn't have a clue, until it was undeniably staring me in the face. A small section contained the photograph of a counsellor based at my GP surgery. It described who she was and who she was able to help. I can't remember the exact criteria she listed, but I know that it resonated with me that day.

I suddenly realised that there was a piece of the puzzle in my hand. I'd been given something tantamount to an oxygen supply after prolonged smoke inhalation. I felt that there was a chance I might breathe again, despite not having a clue how to go about it. I'd never even considered paying to talk to someone before. I'd never imagined that I would want or need to expose all my raw, unpolished, and unattractive vulnerabilities to a complete stranger, with the expectation that they would 'fix' me. But suddenly, in that moment, I knew I had never needed to do that more.

I was lucky. I had friends—incredible, wonderful humans who would listen and give advice, sticking plasters, and hugs. I knew they would extol my finer virtues and paint a convincing picture of what my future might hold...a future that was apparently worth fighting for. But something told me that I also needed someone impartial—someone equipped with qualifications and what I desperately hoped would be a miracle cure.

That was my first experience with counselling and exploring my mental health, but it wasn't my last. That doesn't mean it was a waste of time or that I'm beyond help. It changed my life at the time and opened my eyes to the fact that my mental health is real and it's everything.

Counselling was the proof I needed that I was strong enough to rebuild myself. It also provided the realisation that healing isn't intended to be a solo endeavour. When life propels you into a mental abyss, there's never any shame in reaching out to someone to aid your rescue and recovery...whatever circumstances led you there or however frequently help is needed. My mindset was: why drown when someone is offering to share their lifeboat?

When you're at your lowest point and you've made the decision not to remain there, the only action you can take is to rise up. It isn't meant to be easy. It starts with the realisation that you're in pain but you have the strength and desire to move through it to a more bearable and brighter place, one step at a time. There will be days and moments where you feel as though you can't put one foot in front of the other. But they'll be followed by days and moments where you feel as though you can walk unaided and ultimately stand tall again.

If you get knocked off your feet one day, by an unwelcome or unexpected memory or an emotional response to something or someone you encounter, that's okay. We wake up, we step up, and we do the best we can to believe the smile on our faces. To enjoy the moments we're in and to advocate for our future. There will be moments when we're forced to remember why we began our journey and the pieces and places before it. Something must be broken before it can be repaired. A glow stick must be snapped before it can shine. Any number of triggers can cause wounds to reopen and cracks to come back to the surface. Healing is a verb, which requires us to be present in the present, as active participants of the process.

The smell of an aftershave reminding you of a lost relative. A song from a time that left you behind stinging in your ears and catching in your throat. The sight of a possession belonging to a loved one, who did the unthinkable and walked away, causing your eyes to overflow. The evocative taste of food from a childhood that starved you of affection; crippling your stomach and your soul. The feel of bare, exposed skin, once cradled by a wedding band, leaving you raw, blistered and bruised. All of these experiences remind us that the healing journey can be a sudden, multi-sensory assault on our subconscious.

I believe time does heal. It doesn't come with a prescription pad, starting gun, a finishing date circled on a calendar or a barrel-load of celebratory ticker tape, though. The process is silent, with no fanfare or glamour. It takes its time, allowing us to feel, live through and overcome each moment. One milestone and emotion at a time; time after time. Perhaps we never entirely get past the pain. Perhaps our end point is us adjusting, accepting, and moving forward to a more purposeful and positive kind of peace than we managed the day before. Perhaps time allows us to experience life with more awareness, strength, and gratitude—with the potential for second chances, healing, hope, and happiness.

Labels

If truth be told,
labels can be bought and sold.
Conspicuously consumed
within identity tombs,
by a nation
on the brink of starvation,
hungry for an identity,
whatever that may be.
Can we recognise our reflection
as the tides change direction
in the vast sea
of equal opportunity,
lapping into inequity?
Where we decide
the label we will wear with pride,
perhaps visibly
to some degree,
the label of our choosing,
adorned with the scars and bruising
acquired along the way.

I suppose no one promised it would be easy.

We window shop that which another has,
with eyes akin to the hue of their grass.
Labels are acquired wisely
or frivolously,

depending upon your point of view.
I'll do me, you do you.
Even to this day,
it's a myth to say
that the stagnation
of our imagination
is the only barrier that we face
in the race
to turn the table
and wear the label
we believe to be
our destiny.

We don't always get to choose
if we win or lose.
Maybe I'll have to let it go,
but more than you will ever know,
my heart breaks for the title it won't bear
and the label I'll never own.

I remember once being stood in a queue for the buffet at a party. I think I was in my early twenties. I've always hated the social awkwardness of buffets. You inevitably find yourself queuing up for food whilst trying to select options that won't get stuck in your teeth or end up down your front. You're painfully aware that you can't double-back on yourself if you've missed something good behind you, as

Labels

you try not to take too much or drop your (typically paper) plate. All the while, you're reaching for something at the far end of the table that requires coordination and at least one utensil. You're conscious of those around you, who may or may not be attempting to engage you in polite small talk, as you all unwittingly play an impromptu game of Twister with your various limbs across and around the condiments. That may just be my experience. Anyway, I was stood in the queue, contemplating the scene and the task before me, whilst conversing with a woman I didn't know from Adam. She asked me if I was with someone, romantically speaking. I replied that I was single. I told her this in the same tone and manner as if I were telling her the time or my choice of sandwich filling, yet her response was one of apparent disappointment, shock, horror, and pity. I remember the pity the most. She looked at me as one might look at an animal with a missing limb as she said, 'Oh, never mind. There's still time for you.' I don't really recall what I was most shocked by at the time: the fact a stranger had taken it upon herself to enquire about my relationship status in the first place or the way my single status was akin to a contagious or terminal disease. Yes, I was then, as I am today, a single person. In all honesty, the years in-between, when I was 'attached', didn't provide the happily-ever-after ending I'd imagined and coveted. So why was she feeling sorry for me? Why have I so often felt sorry for myself because I have the label of 'single', rather than 'girlfriend', 'fiancée', 'wife' or simply 'taken'—like an item on display, but with a 'sold' sticker adorning the third finger of my left hand?

Have you ever noticed how our brains seem wired (or socially conditioned, perhaps) to absorb and retain a negative label or criticism rather than a positive label or compliment? If you were to receive 99 compliments and one insult, it's highly likely that the one insult would echo louder and longer through your subconscious mind than all of the compliments combined. From my own experience, I can recall almost every derogatory comment I've ever received with painful accuracy. The loving compliments tend to shrink into the shadows of my memory. They require me to actively recall them, usually as a result of negative memories plaguing my confidence. I'd be surprised if I was the only one affected by this, and that's something I really want to address in this chapter. Our worth is not defined by anyone else's assumptions or perceptions about us. No one else has the right to put a label on us, with the intention or potential to put us in a box and make us feel small due to their judgements.

I recently had a conversation with a woman who was sat outside a shop in my local town centre. She had called me (well, anyone) over to ask if her oversized hooped earrings looked wonky or daft. Apparently, someone had been to Primark and bought them for her and she'd used them to pierce her own ears. She asked me my name and she told me hers. She told me she was an alcoholic and that she'd used the money she'd gathered from begging to buy herself some sunglasses. She asked me if they looked cute. During this conversation, which must have lasted all of five minutes, so much information was shared. I realised afterwards how many labels she'd used—silently and verbally: *alcoholic, self-harmer, single, lesbian, attractive.*

When I looked at her, I didn't see her self-appointed labels (although her arms bore the etchings of one chapter of her story, which may or may not have been the most recent or painful). Instead, I saw a woman with different but equally poignant labels: *human, fallible, lost, lonely, honest.*

I saw a woman with a name, a story, a past, a voice, and a desire to connect with someone, anyone, however briefly, just to remind herself she was alive. She wanted to be seen and heard. She wanted to talk about fashion and books. She gave me a compliment. She thanked me for taking the time to talk to her. She asked me questions. She didn't want food, she wanted alcohol. Maybe her hunger came from somewhere deeper to reach than her stomach. Maybe the drink would have been more numbing than nutritious. Maybe that was what she needed. I think she needed a lot, i.e. to be validated through an interaction with another person, to have choices, to have respect, to have hope, to have a drink. She was a stranger with a story to tell, but she could have been any one of us.

Our world is seemingly obsessed with labels, identity, what or who we identity with or as; obsessed with status and presentation. Maybe we need to take the time to see beyond the skin-deep labels and the make-up, which help to create the make-believe and see the person that lies beneath it all. I suspect we're not that different beneath the surface, whatever our surface looks like. If I'd asked that woman, 'Do you know what has happened to you?', I wonder how long it would have taken her to answer that, even to herself. I wonder how painful an experience that might have been for her.

If you were to sit alone with your labels and silently name them all, what would your list look like? How many of those labels did you choose through desire and dedication? How many were handed down to you as a hereditary heirloom? How many were conceived from accidental or coincidental twists of fate? How many were forced upon you? How much gratitude do you attach to each one? Which bring you pride, and which are attributed to your regret or shame? How many of these labels are kind, truthful or accurate representations of you? Sometimes, we don't get a choice. Some labels will always bear the hallmark of resentment rather than pride. But no label tells the whole story, or even the absolute truth, of who we are, what we've lived through, where we've been, where we might end up, or all that we're capable of.

Like a traditional Russian stacking doll, we each have a visible presence—a physical profile—that we present to the world as a descriptive billboard. It details our more evident features and labels. Yet, like the title of a book, it may conceal ambiguous undertones. Others may guess at our age, our gender, our dress size, and our profession, based on what society has conditioned them to interpret with the naked eye. But they won't know how kind each of those years have been to us, how comfortable we feel within the skin we're in or the emotional weight of that number on the label of our clothes. They may see an expectant mother, but not the circumstances or emotional journey she's experienced to wear that label. They may see a visible health condition or a sensory impairment, but they won't be able to read the invisible subtitles beneath. They may see the presence of a wedding ring, but not the bereavement that may have followed, bringing an entirely unwelcome label in its wake.

Concealed beneath the outer shell, we carry the less obvious and more accurate stories behind the chapter headings. These form the narrative only those who take the time to peel back the layers and read between the lines can ever begin to know us by. Studies have shown that 93% of our communication is non-verbal and inferred rather than heard. I would suggest a similar proportion of our labels and narrative lies beneath the surface; visible to only a select few—one of which may, with enough time and introspection, be ourselves. Those who defy society's expectations for judgement and categorisation, and those who choose to see a little deeper and know a little more, become our people. They become our secret-keepers, our advocates, and our cheerleaders. They see the real within our reality. These people, through character and choice, are often blind and indifferent to our labels.

At our inner core are all the things that defy labels and which persistently, proudly, and painfully reside within us. Our childhood experiences, adverse or otherwise, and our inner voice, with its daily dialogue, are all the faceless foundations upon which all other more prominent experiences and labels are built.

Several years ago, I had a realisation; in part, courtesy of Denzel Washington. I was sat in a primary school assembly hall as a thirty-four-year-old with so many insecurities and perceived failures under my belt. I was on the cusp of embarking upon one of the most terrifying and life-affirming journeys of my life. It was day one of my PGCE training. The head teacher at the school where I would be based for a period of my practical teaching practice played us all—seasoned professionals and novices alike—a video of Denzel delivering a commencement speech to graduates at the University of Pennsylvania on May 16th, 2011. It was entitled 'Fall Forward'. Perhaps you know it. If you don't, I'd urge you to go on YouTube and watch it in its entirety. It was one of the most profound and poignant things I'd ever heard, and I absorbed every word like a cactus taking in water. I told friends about it, I embraced it, I felt empowered by it, and ultimately, at the moments when I needed it the most, I forgot about it—until now. Your failures don't define you. They make all future successes possible. They spur you on. They make you stronger, more determined, more committed to your goals and your development. They make you more three-dimensional as a person. They make you human.

Denzel addressed the audience of expectant students, who were on the brink of their next adventure and ensuing life choices. He spoke about Thomas Edison being known and celebrated for creating the light bulb. However, he suggested that no one remembers, documents or discusses the 1000 attempts that resulted in failure and which preceded his breakthrough. He shared that, at the start of his own career, he'd repeatedly failed at auditions. Rather than giving up and falling back on something different, safer or more predictable, he persevered. He practised, and he prayed. Falling back wasn't a concept he bought into. Instead, he preferred the mindset of falling forward into something he believed in and could see coming. He learned and grew from every failure, every missed opportunity, every deviation in direction, and every attempt that failed to yield success.

I personally wish that our education system invested and believed in the principles of teaching children to accept and embrace their fails—i.e. their first attempts in learning—as much as they believe in targets, tests, and statistics. Should children not be encouraged to see themselves with positivity, as the developing, imperfect children they are and the adults they'll become? They're each filled with promise, potential, and the strength from having tried, which is surely better than allowing a fear of failure to prevent them from never trying at all. One of the most soul-destroying moments in my training came during a Year 4 standardised test, in which eight- and nine-year-olds, during a global and life-altering pandemic, were required to answer questions from a test paper without any adult assistance. The children were tearful, angry, frustrated, and scared. They were worried about making a mistake and getting it wrong. One naturally bright boy found it an unsettling experience. Where numbers are concerned, he excelled. He understood them, they made sense to him, and he usually got the answer right. With one particular question on this test, he kept asking me for help and clarification. I apologetically repeated that I could only read the question for him, yet we both knew that that was no help to him at all. Children are used to raising their hand, once they've overcome any embarrassment or reluctance to do so, to ask for help and understanding and they trust that their teacher will do their best to give it in one form or another. Yet all I was doing in that situation was watching a conscientious and confused child crumble in front of me, as he did his best not to fail that question and anyone else's expectations of him —including his own.

I couldn't tell him in that moment that, in reality, a month, a year or a decade down the line, this moment would be both forgotten and irrelevant to the outcome of his life. Or that this moment played no part in defining his identity, his worth or his abilities. I wanted to say all of those things, as I'd been in that same position myself so many times. I'd mentally tortured and berated myself for saying or doing the wrong thing in a situation; for being too much of some things and not enough of others. For worrying myself sick over an innocent mistake or something outside of my control. For letting others down or being less than perfect, which, of course, is exactly what we all are by design, rather than by defect. I was never taught at school how to appreciate myself and my efforts, how to develop emotional resilience or how to rise above unrealistic expectations or damaging labels.

I've had to learn the following nuggets of gold throughout decades of my life:

- It's okay to not have it all figured out by a certain age, milestone, moment or marker
- Success is personal and you don't owe anyone else an interpretation, justification or apology for what this looks like for you
- It's better to try, learn, and grow than never to try at all
- Self-conviction and self-love are two of the greatest achievements and successes you can experience in life.

Personally, I agree with Denzel Washington. Never stop trying, learning, growing, redefining, and reimagining yourself. You don't want the ghosts of missed opportunities and unrealised dreams, possibilities, and achievements assembling around your death bed, in accusatory judgement because you turned your back on them when you had the chance. His speech concluded with the words, *'The chances you take, the people you meet, the people you love, the faith that you have, that's what's going to define you. Whenever you fall throughout life, remember this: fall forward.'*

The way we speak to ourselves matters, as much as the decision we make to breathe. The words and labels we use, to ourselves and about ourselves, carry so much weight that they have the power to knock us off our feet and potentially paralyse us. They can cause us to detest ourselves, to the point that we offer discounts on our worth to those we interact with, work with, live with, and whom we're intimate with. This affects and determines our relationships with others, until a self-fulfilling prophecy emerges. At the most severe, we're treated by others with the contempt we feel for ourselves. Or, at the equally unacceptable end of the spectrum, their attitude towards us reinforces, rather than challenges, our own.

For every label I proudly have—daughter, niece, cousin, friend, aunty, godmother, to name a few—it's the label of what I am not that weighs most invisibly, yet heavily, around my heart: a mother. One of my friends so poignantly and casually coined the phrase to me many years ago: always the godmother, never the mother. This hit me around the face with more brutality than a wet, concrete fish. I know he will not remember that conversation any more than he remembers what he had for breakfast that day or what colour his socks were—but I remember it with crystal clarity.

Labels

That's the thing about labels...they attach themselves to you like a second skin and become the things you're known by, judged on, and are answerable to. They lie with you in the darkness and sit with you in the most crowded space.

In April 2020, The Guardian published a report conducted by Office Angels. It found that 70% of office workers would prefer a more pompous and prominent sounding job title to a pay rise. Admittedly, this was a few years before the cost-of-living crisis hit. Perhaps fewer people asked today would be so willing to exchange the ability to heat their homes for a fancier email signature, but it says a hell of a lot about the significance we place on labels in a professional context. These job titles may do little to inflate our bank accounts, but they're seemingly credited with the ability to expand our status, social standing, credibility, and worth. Says who? Who gets to decide that a 'chief imagination officer' is a more worthy title for a 'creative assistant'? Who decides whether a 'single' person should be pitied or put up for public comment or scrutiny? Who's in a position to say that anyone's worth should be defined, measured or judged by any label, self-chosen or otherwise?

Do I know who I am? I'm beginning to. Do I

want to live this way? No, not completely. But I am, just like you are, so much more than any label attached to me. We're all infinitely more than the skin we're in.

You are a whole person, not one fragmented piece that can provide or reduce your worth. You are enough, irrespective of anyone else's perspective. It can often take a lifetime to accept or truly believe this for, and about, ourselves. This acceptance, like our evolution as fully functioning humans, is a daily work in progress, but the fact you're still trying means you're not quitting. You're refusing to give up on yourself or your future. You're striving for the life you want to live. If you're falling, which you will do on a regular basis because you're human, you're falling forward—with hope, optimism, and determination.

My hope is that, if nothing else, this book allows you to view yourself as you are: a whole, complex, and valuable human. Regardless of your starting point, your journey or your destination, you and your reflection will always be enough. I understand that, whilst this is the most important thing we will ever learn, we need to learn it through experience and believe it from our hearts. Me telling you you're enough may not be a life-affirming or altering revelation for you. You may not personally be

there yet—which is okay, as yet is the most important word in all of this. I just hope you can repeat these words back to yourself on a daily basis until you're able to believe them.
You are enough.

One concept that children are increasingly becoming exposed to is having a growth mindset. This is ultimately the affirmation that, whilst you may not be able to do or achieve something yet, by acknowledging the yet, you're recognising that this is not the end of the experience, the learning or the journey. Just like Thomas Edison, all your failed attempts will one day reward you with success. If you look upon those mistakes as character-building, memory making, and resolve-strengthening, they will become your gold.

I can't do this...yet.
I'm not who or where I want to be...yet.
This is not the life I want to live...yet.

It's never too late to learn and practise this. Maybe the more we teach this—in classrooms, in homes, in the workplace, in the silence that hosts our thoughts and our reflections—the more we will see that our journey teaches us more than the destination (potentially) ever could. Persistence and pride can be some of our greatest successes. Practice conceives strength of character and determination. Every curve in the road, every deviation, every backbreaking moment before our big break and our happily-right-now, is our achievement—just as much as the lightbulb moment that may be our final perceived legacy.

Can you add a 'yet' to the end of your life's current blockades, in order to provide a different perspective or outcome?

Your shoes don't define you; it's the way that you wear them

May I introduce you to the person before you;
the one you don't see?
May I use words unspoken
to tell you my story?
May you look beyond the surface
of all that I have become.
May you see that this transition in me
is as unavoidable as the setting of the sun.
May you look with eyes devoid of judgement
and view me with the same patience and love
as I have looked upon you, my child,
my blessing from above.
I have raised you good
and I have raised you well,
so I ask you to sit with me for a while
so my story I can tell.
For I was not always so helpless,
but it seems that you forgot,
when you decided that I was defined,
by all the things that I am not.
I am not the patient you see
sat before you in this chair.
I am the mother who bathed you daily
with water, love and care.
I am not the shell
of the person I used to be.

*I am the parent who caught you when you fell
and kissed your injured knee.
I am not the woman in room 409
who forgets when and how to eat.
I am the person who always picked you up
and put you back upon your feet.
I am not the figure of fragility
lying in this bed,
with time having taken over my body
and this condition taking over my head.
I am so much more than all of this;
so much more than the imperfect picture that
you see.
I am strong. I am beautiful. I am proud.
I am me.
I am the soothing warmth in winter.
I am your favourite Sunday roast.
I am every bedtime story.
I am your breakfast dippy eggs and regimented
soldier toast.
I am your trusted confidante
when your eyes are wet and raw.
I am the narrator of your story
and all that came before.
I am so much more than all of this,
so much more than all you forgot I could be;
A woman. A wife. Your mother.
I am every shade of me.
I am the sweet sound of your laughter,*

*I am every tear that you cry.
I am the peace that comforts you before you fall asleep.
I am every butterfly.*

When I turned thirty, I had an age-related mental meltdown. I didn't just dip my toe in denial, I bathed in it daily. If I didn't acknowledge it, it wasn't happening. Not on my watch. I refused to believe I was entering my fourth decade without having achieved the things on my life's tick-list. The milestones and accomplishments I'd decided from a young age were a case of not if they were going to happen, but when. That *when* was rapidly slipping through my fingers, out of my control, against my will, leaving me with a residual ache in my stomach and my body weight in regret and resentment. It turns out that life had other ideas. It left me unable to move past my inability to tick off the achievements and milestones I thought were guaranteed, solely because I wanted them enough. For a painfully long time, I saw myself as inadequate, broken, and purposeless. I saw everything that I wasn't —the invisible taunting emptiness, rather than the visible, tangible things I was. I was consumed by an overwhelming sense of not being enough, because I wasn't living the life I wanted...the life that seemed mockingly visible yet irrefutably out of reach.

I want to use this chapter to encourage and support you to see yourself above your condition. To see your abilities above your limitations and to see your haves above your have-nots. To see your strength above your pain, so others will be encouraged to view you in the same way, i.e. the way you deserve to be seen. Trust me when I say, from experience, I know that's easier said than done. It is, however, the thing that will save you from a lifetime of feeling less, of feeling judged, and feeling bruised and scarred from the stick you beat yourself with.

If life causes your memories to fade or your words start to fail you. If your abilities, mobility or independence become compromised. If your choices become limited or if your health begins to decline. If life causes your appearance to change, your confidence to falter, your life to become unrecognisable or your future to become uncertain, it can utterly paralyse you with fear, devastation, anger, and resentment. It can strip you of your dignity, heighten your defences, test the depth and permanence of your relationships, and knock you off your feet. Every day can feel like a battle you're ill-prepared to fight in, let alone win. You may see yourself as less than all you've ever been, as your reflection asks you who you are, if you're not all that you were. Whether you've been diagnosed with a medical condition or your change is brought about through ageing, there is, perhaps, an unavoidable period of mourning for the life you lived before, and an uncomfortable adjustment to the future you face. Please remember, whilst circumstances, capabilities and outlooks change, you remain the constant in a sea of change. You are a human being: an intricate arrangement of atoms that combine perfectly to form the body that supports and sustains you. Your body adapts to all it endures and carries you through each second of your existence—regardless of how painful, challenging or impossible it may seem. You're an abundance of emotions, memories, skills, and experiences, contained within a miraculous and unique life-sustaining shell. This perfectly imperfect exterior can and will change, like an emotive chameleon adapting to its environment. You are as you as you have ever been, and that's the indisputable truth that runs through your core, like a message in a stick of rock.

A diagnosis can feel like a social stigma, a door closing on inclusivity or a distorted mirror. It can become a silent assassin you need to keep one step ahead of, as you constantly search for a cure or a means to disempower it. Receiving a diagnosis can feel like an undetonated bomb in our hands and our minds. There's the potential that absolutely everything will change, with immediate and devastating effect. We almost convince ourselves that we've taken on an entirely new identity, after being given a condition we didn't ask for or a diagnosis we cannot pronounce or fathom. It may dent our resolve and cause a fault line in our immunity, but it cannot ever touch our character, our personality, and our intrinsic worth. We possibly all have some experience of a decline in health–sudden or prolonged—that has affected ourselves or someone we know and love. This may cause us to automatically consider a worst-case scenario. We may mentally enable the condition to become bigger than the person.

Since 2020, I have been given one diagnosis that I was convinced I was too young to realistically receive, another that I was paranoid would ultimately lead to a decline in my sight and a third that I can just about pronounce. I will, however, have the rest of my life to become aquatinted with its pronunciation and symptoms. With each diagnosis, I took myself out of the moment I was in and envisaged a future down the line that I had no control over, but which I was predicting would be physically and emotionally challenging. None of these conditions are, so far, particularly advanced or catastrophic, but, in a typically human way, I catastrophised them and took myself down a proverbial prognosis rabbit hole. I compared myself to other people I knew. I took some relief and comfort from those with similar experiences. I also looked at others who had no health conditions, concerns or ailments (that I knew of) and wished I was in their shoes. Eventually, a healthy and rational perspective kicked in and I realised that things could be worse. I can contemplate the view from the bridge when I eventually come to cross it.

I've also seen people I love, as they've journeyed towards, over, and past that metaphorical bridge, and I've realised how difficult and unfair that journey was for them. As you go through life, you love more people, you live more years and experience more threats to your youth, your health, and your sense of self. A fear of all that cannot be predicted or prevented seems to become an increasingly constant companion.

Life may change your appearance, your outlook or your capabilities, but you're more than any combination of symptoms or conditions—however debilitating or difficult they may be to live with. You are still you, with the strength, personality, heart, and soul you've always been armed with.

Do you know what has happened to you?

Your appearance is unique to you, as are the metaphorical shoes you wear to move through life. No one but you will ever experience what it's like to see through your eyes. Others cannot feel the pain and sensations within your body or experience their intensity as they ebb and flow. No one but you will live with and alongside your thoughts, as they both celebrate and berate you, minute to minute. Your shoes don't define you; it's the way you wear them that matters. Keep moving onwards, with pride and purpose, no matter what the blisters or obstacles. Don't be embarrassed or afraid to slow down, to pause, and to show the pain when it comes. Those who care about you will always stop to walk alongside you, to offer you shelter and company, or take you by the hand and navigate the landscape with you.

In November 2022, the Office for National Statistics (ONS) detailed data from the 2021 census, in relation to the ageing population of England and Wales. It drew comparisons between the results of 2021 and the previous census a decade earlier. Over 11 million people in 2021 were aged 65 or older, compared to nine million in 2011, which included over 500,000 people who were at least 90 years of age. Regardless of the number of years they'd been alive and whatever age bracket they fell into, that data does not represent soulless, inconsequential figures. It provides a statistical snapshot of millions of individual people, who have lived varied and meaningful lives and touched many others. They could be you, your relative, your friend or neighbour or the stranger you interact with for a moment in time. They are all of us, just with a few extra years of experience under their belts and a more visible history etched across their skin.

A 75-year-old respondent broke down the dividing barriers between the generations when she said, 'I don't feel old. Inside, I am still me. Older people are just people who have lived longer than others.' When put that way, surely those 11 million people had been given the ultimate gift of time. They were fortunate enough to have survived all they'd encountered during more than six decades, each with a different narrative but all with the same level of enoughness. To grow older isn't nature's punishment. It's a priceless gift, denied to so many who are taken too brutally, too suddenly, and too soon.

Your age isn't a number to dread, deny or dodge like a bullet. Your age is the number of sunsets you've witnessed, the number of mornings in which you've awoken to live and experience another day and the number of holidays you've enjoyed. It's the number of photographs you've taken, the number of friends you've made, and the number of 'I love yous' you've said and received. It's the number of smiles you've shared, the number of lives you've touched, and the number of memories you've made.

Imagine your life as a suitcase. It starts off brand-new, shiny, vast, empty of contents but full of potential. With each passing day that accumulates into years, you store memories, people, experiences and feelings inside it... keepsakes of a life lived. As time passes, your suitcase becomes heavier, weathered, and more fragile. Eventually, it buckles under the weight of its precious contents; your heirlooms to share and your legacy to leave. Only by being alive are you able to continue to fill your suitcase. Whilst every experience may not be positive, they sit alongside better ones; this helps cushion the blow a little, and they give you the incentive and strength to fight for more. Some people's suitcases are never given the opportunity to become as full and worn as they were intended to be. Our own suitcases, our own lives, should never be taken for granted, discarded or wasted.

Person-first language emphasises the person before the condition or the difficulty they're living with and, in my opinion, this is a positive thing. You are the person holding your suitcase. Your experiences, traumas, health conditions, and circumstances are simply the contents of the suitcase you're carrying. They're not bigger than you and they don't define you. They can be put down at any time whilst you pause, take a breath, and enjoy the experience of being a person that indisputably matters.

During my teacher training, we were told that, once you've met a child with autism, you've met one child with autism. That seemingly obvious statement is actually one of the most enlightening pieces of information I received. It served to remind me that, once you've met one person with any background, label, condition or set of experiences, you've met one person. They're not a statistic, stereotype, sufferer or problem to be solved. The same is also true for you.

Do not see yourself as old. See yourself as

privileged to have a suitcase you're still able to fill. Don't see your afflictions or ailments; see your strength that keeps you going. Don't meet your altered appearance with disgust or defiance; embrace the body that adapts as it was designed to do in order to sustain you. Don't respond to your reflection with negativity, regret, and attempts to turn back time; react with appreciation for the opportunity to showcase a different layer of your beauty. Whatever you see as you look into the eyes of the person before you—a fellow human or your own reflection—always look hard and deep enough to see the whole, intricate person, rather than their more visible struggles, shell or shame. Try to read, hear, and appreciate the story they don't share aloud. They're still there, concealed under years of living and searching for enoughness, in a world that judges them for all the ways they've changed, whilst being blind to all that has never changed.

Whoever you are, whatever has happened to you, wherever your shoes take you, and whatever condition they're in, you're always so much more than the cover the world sees. You are the whole damn book.

The black dog's bark

The black dog's bark
echoes into the abyss
yet manages to miss
the ears of the deaf and the immune
who hear instead
the sweeter tune
of the hummingbird or the lark
but they are not to blame
as a rose by any other name
is still exactly that
and who can blame those
whose eyes only allow them to see
what is in plain sight?
The black dog's bark
is muffled and muzzled
by the void
which is devoid
of the natural light
that belongs to another world
and another view
but which, from time to time,
permeates through
the darkness
to remind you of a world
that you once knew
but which you counter has
forgotten you

*as it taunts you with
the reflection of a stranger
who mirrors the appearance
of someone familiar
behind the mask
of a strategically placed smile
which extends for a mile
and yet leads nowhere at all.*

A wonderful friend once asked me, 'How's your mental health?' No one had ever asked me such a pertinent question before. It felt so raw, refreshing, and unexpected that I didn't really know how to respond. I didn't realise or fully appreciate it at the time, but it was a gift. It seems a very weighted question when we consider that, for so many of us, we may have never had the reason or opportunity to question or understand what the term 'mental health' might mean. If we do, it's usually when we've reached a point of crisis, rather than conversation. It seems important to understand the term and the implications of mental health at the stable door, so to speak, rather than whilst restraining or retreating from a bolting horse.

The World Health Organisation (WHO) defines mental health as:
A state of mental wellbeing that enables people

to cope with the stresses of life, realise their abilities, learn well and work well and contribute to their community. It is an integral component of health and wellbeing that underpins our individual and collective abilities to make decisions, build relationships and shape the world we live in.

Let's consider our overall health as a tree. Rooted intrinsically and universally within each of us, our mental health is just one branch of that life-sustaining tree—alongside our emotional, spiritual, physical, cognitive, neurological, visual, and auditory health. This tree needs constant and committed nurturing. If one branch becomes weakened, damaged or vulnerable, the body as a whole feels the effects. We need to recognise our mental health as being our life-blood, our identity, and our basic human right. It's something we each possess, but few of us recognise, appreciate or know how to nurture, strengthen or repair it.

As a society, we ask each other 'How are you?', often expecting very little in the way of detail or the actual truth. When I started work in a previous job, I soon realised that 'Alright' was actually just a greeting and a statement; it wasn't necessarily accompanied by an invisible question mark at the end. Yet I interpreted one as being there, and I would reply with, 'Fine, thanks. You?' This turned out to be a completely unnecessary and slightly embarrassing response, as the other person would have often walked off after throwing their casual greeting my way. I realised that people don't always want the truth—especially not a convoluted or honest version—even when a question has been asked and a response is socially acceptable.

How often have you been asked "how are you?" and been socially aware before you answer that this is often a perfunctory greeting or question, with the purpose of being polite, passing the time of day, or performing a social norm or nicety? It's hardly ever a result of someone actually wanting to hear about your sleep deprivation, financial worries, holiday plans or your latest health condition, etc. More often than not, we respond with, 'I'm fine, thanks. How are you?' This is taken at face value and a similar sentiment is shared in response, until the conversation moves in another direction or it comes to a natural end.

I did an introductory-level 'counselling concepts' course many years ago. I remember the tutor discussing the notion of greeting someone with a polite and perfunctory 'How are you?' She suggested that the trite and yet safe response of 'I'm FINE, thanks' is actually a mnemonic for 'I'm Fucked-up, Insecure, Neurotic and Emotional, thanks for asking. Now what are you going to do with that information?' I imagine that 'Fed-up, Irritated, Nervous and Exhausted' would equally suffice; adjust and amend the mnemonic to suit your mood and preference. Whichever emotions you attach to it, the point is, telling someone you are 'FINE' can be tantamount to covering the mouth of a volcano with a botanical garden. On the surface, it's aesthetically pleasing and supports the equilibrium of the local environment, reassuring everyone who passes by that all is well and as it should be. Beneath the surface, however, an internal hell could be simmering. Maybe, as a race and a society, we've become conditioned to look without seeing and to listen without hearing, i.e. taking things at face value until the truth erupts, one way or another. Maybe next time we see a beautiful landscape, we could question the foundations it rests upon. Maybe next time someone tells us they're fine, we could look a little deeper to read between the lines and hear the words they may not be saying.

Duvet days can be an indulgent tonic. They contribute to our diet of self-care, encouraging us to take the time to wrap ourselves in the warmth and security of a grown-up comfort blanket, and to focus on something enjoyable and manageable in the here and now. That could be mentally engaging with a Sudoku puzzle or passively watching reruns of a favourite box set. Duvet days can be a luxurious treat, a temporary vacation from the demands of reality and the opportunity to mentally check-in with ourselves and ask, *'What do I need today? Why do I feel this way? Who am I and how do I feel in this moment, when I'm alone and answerable to no one but myself? What are my heart and mind telling me, and are they in agreement with each other?'*

Duvet days can be a warming hot chocolate on a bitter winter's night, a hug when we need soothing or a pause button on life when it's at its most frantic. They can allow us to recharge, reset, and recover. Duvet days can be the answer to a passing problem. However, duvet days themselves become a problem when they occur one after another, like a trail of breadcrumbs leading to an ultimately grim destination. When duvet days become the foundation of our week and an emotional crutch, rather than a temporary plaster, this is when they can become suffocating. This is when we're at our most vulnerable and this can be why we stop breathing. When duvet days become our norm and isolation becomes our safety net, we're retreating from the reality that provides the people, the clarity, the moments, and the opportunities that can strengthen and heal us. By encasing ourselves in the darkness and safety of the duvet, we're also enveloping our emotions in the darkness that nestles within the duvet—alongside us and within us—as an oppressive sleeping companion. Within the silence our minds speak the loudest, with nothing to counteract the often-destructive noise. We cocoon ourselves from reality, from stress, from our reflection, and from our distorted view of everything within and beyond us. The cocoon begins to suffocate us as much as it shelters us.

Inside a chrysalis, a caterpillar's body digests itself from the inside out. The same juices it once used to digest its food, it now uses to break down its own body. The transformation only becomes miraculous and beautiful once it's complete, when the new body has formed, and it has the strength and capacity to emerge into the world anew. Until it figures out a way to escape its environment, it remains neither what it was, nor what it has become. The caterpillar's self-mutilation in pursuit of progression, of development, of change, will have been futile if it cannot ultimately escape into the light. Nothing survives or thrives in darkness (with the exception of bats and glow-worms). Nothing can live in the shadows of the past. My point is: a spoonful of sugar may help life become a less bitter pill to swallow, but when you can't taste life without an accompanying sweet anaesthetic, you become desensitised and fall into in a diabetic coma, minus your teeth.

The caterpillar must rely on itself in order to leave its previous body and old life behind; to break down its physical defences and for its transformative state to be complete. Whilst writing this, it struck me what a terrifying, lonely, and claustrophobic environment a chrysalis must be. Granted, I am perceiving and describing it from a human perspective. It's unlikely that an insect would have the same emotional response or awareness to its environment or circumstances as we humans would. I guess, in turn, their experience of metamorphosis is something we'll never fully appreciate or understand. You're not an insect, obviously, but you are fragile, whilst also being capable of miraculous healing. However, much like the caterpillar, that growth and everything that happens leading up to it must start with you making a choice. We have the choice to remain in the physical duvet and its psychological confines or we can break out and emerge past the pain and darkness and take tentative steps towards recovery. When we feel most alone, that's when we need to name our emotions, whatever they may be, and make the bravest decision of all—to reach out in order to break out.

As I mentioned earlier, we all have mental health. Unlike with our physical health, we don't have an inbuilt immune system on high alert 24/7, ready to defend our mind, body, and soul from an onslaught of negative thoughts and stress factors. However, our mental and physical health are intrinsically linked. When one is under attack, the other suffers. A mental illness of any kind, and I cannot stress this enough, is no more of a stigma than a physical illness. Yet the human race appears to have lost the ability to be kind to itself. Instead, it looks upon mental health with eyes that demand to see in order to believe. A lack of visible symptoms does not negate severity. If anything, they heighten the threat, as their detrimental effects can remain undetected for longer, often hidden in plain sight. All mental illnesses, including anxiety and depression, look different for every person who's affected by them. There's no blueprint, mould or stereotype for someone suffering from a mental illness, and no individual, absolute trigger to ignite or exacerbate the symptoms. A person's circumstances, feelings, and coping mechanisms are as unique as they are. When you've met a person with depression or anxiety, you've met only one person with depression or anxiety. They may fall into one category or sit under an umbrella diagnosis, but each one of the approximately 280 million global sufferers of depression will tell a completely unique story. It's up to everyone else to take the time to listen and understand their narrative.

The statistics relating to mental health conditions are truly terrifying. The Priory states that, in England, one in six people—equivalent to approximately 45.8 million adults—report experiencing symptoms for common mental health problems, such as anxiety and depression, in any given week. 25% of people in England—close to 14.1 million adults—said they felt lonely at least some of the time. This is less surprising but quite poignant; data for wellbeing and loneliness was obtained between March 2020 and April 2021. This was perhaps the most physically and emotionally isolating and mentally detrimental period, on a global scale, in generations. Data from Age UK in February 2023 states that 1.4 million people over the age of 65 are lonely. At the opposite end of the age spectrum, the World Health

Organisation detailed in November 2021, that one in seven 10–19-year-olds, globally, experience a mental disorder. It increasingly feels as though mental health has become the elephant in the room. We're all aware of it, but we're reluctant to voice it aloud. If we startle it by naming it or aggravate it by approaching it, we seem to fear that we may cause pandemonium. What the eye can't see the mind can't worry about. And yet, of course, it does. Worry may be akin to sitting in a rocking chair to pass the time. Ultimately, it gets us nowhere, or at least nowhere productive, yet, we all sit in that chair for varying lengths of time, on any typical day, in any given week, throughout our lives. Opportunities to worry are as abundant as the cracks in a crazy-paved path. Any one of them has the potential to trip us up at any given moment, if we're not paying attention or if life takes us unaware. I believe that it's not only the frequency and the severity of the falls we encounter in life that cause damage to our mental health but also our response to them. *Was anyone there to witness the fall, to comment, to help, to make matters better or worse? Did anyone catch you as you fell? Did they notice? Did they care? Did you torturously carry the guilt for the fall yourself, or lay it in anger on anyone else's shoulders?*

How often did your mind replay it? How deep was the wound, and how much strength did it take you to rise again?

Some of the most emotionally-crippling events of my life have been unremarkable in nature. However, I think your level of reaction is dependent upon your prior level of exposure to trauma and pain, and the ACEs or ALEs you've collected and survived along the way. What may cripple you one year may barely leave a scratch the next, depending on what you've lived through and the emotional resilience you develop. Life doesn't tell you the required or acceptable level of pain to feel in any given situation. It doesn't decide the duration of your grief or anger or the level of intensity to your emotions. Nor does it dictate how to navigate trauma, impossible decisions, rejection, loneliness, fear or any of the other feelings that lurk in the shadows, waiting to overwhelm and ambush us when we're at our most vulnerable. And nor should it. No guidebook, no person, no platform or community should decide what emotional reaction any of us have to the things we deal with in life. Emotional reactions don't come in a one-size-fits-all package, and that's something I want to emphasise. No one else can live your life for you. People may hear your stories, but they don't know what was rampaging through your head and your heart as the story played out. You and you alone were in your skin and your shoes at that moment in time. You bear the memories and the scars, the tear stains and the trauma. That's your silent narrative and you don't need to add subtitles for anyone else's benefit. We should, however, all be prepared and equipped to read between the unspoken lines.

Whether you're helping someone else or you're in need of help yourself, please reach out. There's no stigma around making contact with another human being or making a connection in a world that's becoming increasingly virtual and decreasingly empathetic. It's not intrusive to offer help to another person, to extend a hand or to provide validation through an acknowledgment of their presence, if not their pain. It's never weak to ask for or accept help. They say it takes a village to raise a child. Equally, it can take a sole villager to raise someone to their feet, to lead them back to their village and back to themselves. You could be that villager. To leave the duvet or to escape from the cocoon, the desire and the intention need to start from within. Once you realise you're worth the fight —and I promise you that you are—you'll always find someone to become your tribe, to join your tribe, to strengthen your tribe, to fight your corner for you, and to catch you when you fall.

40% of men said they would need to experience thoughts of suicide or self-harm before seeking professional help. Please use your voice and reach out, so that you or anyone you love or encounter can avoid becoming a statistic. Starting a conversation can be heroic. Starting a conversation could change someone's day. Starting a conversation could change a life. You don't need to be an expert or a professional; you just need to be a person that cares enough to offer a safe space, patience, and time to another human. You need to give more than a passing glance and a passive response to someone who may feel invisible, lost, broken or silently suicidal. They may feel everything, or they may feel nothing at all. If you look into the eyes of your reflection or the next person you have an interaction with, I hope you look with care, patience and eyes that see beyond the surface, without judgement or fear. I hope you look with love and I hope love wins.

Below are a few ways to remind yourself of your achievements, your value, and your worth. They work for me in varying degrees; I hope they may do the same for you. Over time, why not add your own self-love strategies?

- **Give yourself a compliment every day, or as often as possible**

It could be based on something you feel you did well.
Something you achieved or overcame.
The way you turned a negative or awkward moment into something more positive.
The difference you were able to make to another person's day or outlook.
Or something more surface level...such as the fact you felt beautiful or confident in an outfit or after trying a new hairstyle or perfume.

Write down one compliment to yourself daily. Store them somewhere safe and read them back when you need a reminder of how much there is to love about yourself.

- **Surround yourself with visual reminders of all that there is to love and celebrate about you and the life you live. These might be:**

Favourite photographs from a time or place when you looked or felt the best, happiest version of yourself, which can be a comfort and inspiration.

A certificate, award or memento from a time when you overcame your own expectations and achieved more than you thought you were capable of. Or when your talent, dedication, blood, sweat, and tears resulted in something you're truly proud of.

- **If you receive a compliment, a gift or something meaningful that comes from a place of love, gratitude or appreciation, keep it close and visible**

These souvenirs will remind you that you matter to others.

You're loved unconditionally for who you are and what you bring to a friendship, a situation or another person.

Others see incredible, positive things in you that draw them to you.

Hopefully, these reminders may help you find the qualities you're loved for by others—so that their love becomes self-love.

- **End each day with forgiveness and kindness towards yourself**

If something didn't go well, if something or someone upset you or your day was harder than most, remind yourself that you showed up, you tried, you learned, and you grew. This is just a part of your story rather than the end of it. A mistake is a bruise, rather than a tattoo. Whatever it is doesn't define you. You're enough as you are. You're deserving of love, irrespective of what you've dealt with in the day or the way you responded to whatever you encountered.

- **Write yourself an honest letter**

Discuss your feelings, aspirations, and relationships. Be unflinchingly raw and address the issues and emotions that you might not be brave enough to name or say aloud, but which you feel are the most significant. Lay blame sparingly. Blaming others solves nothing and blaming yourself serves as self-sabotage. It's a stitch in your tapestry, and to unpick it could cause your perspective, positivity, and present to unravel. Acknowledging its existence and impact can be cathartic. Unburden your heart and mind and let your narrative flow through your pen, in a silent and private outpouring of a life lived and the imprint it's left. It's up to you if you choose to keep the letter afterwards. If you do, please don't be tempted to use it as a stick to beat yourself with, but rather as a quiet reflection and introspection, hopefully laced with love and forgiveness. Let it be whatever you need it to be. If a future version of yourself does read it back, I hope it will be with an element of gratitude for the highs you experienced and pride in yourself for the challenges that you overcame.

- **Control your circle of influences**

The people we surround ourselves with have a direct influence on how we talk to, and about, ourselves. Take note of those who build you up and those who tear you down, verbally or physically. Separate the tonic from the toxic. Your power lies in what you pay attention to, how you respond to others and the talk that you listen to.

The hero behind the mask

A hero is not defined by a costume
of Lycra and neon tights.
Instead, they wear their heart on their sleeve
and every day is a different fight.

Friends dance with wolves,
whilst foes masquerade in wool.
Hiding in plain sight;
attempting to break the beautiful.

The world looks upon the hero
with eyes that do not see.
Blind to the potential
concealed behind their identity.

Memories of the past are their kryptonite.
They didn't think it would end this way.
Blindsided by the twists of fate,
which haunt them every day.

Their demons lie below the surface,
feeding upon their insecurities.
One day our hero is positive;
the next they're on their knees.

They draw strength from fragility.
Their smile is their disguise,

shielding them from exposure,
to the pain behind their eyes.

But that is not to say that
strength relies upon deception,
as the mask they wear
can be their greatest shield of protection.

Ask any hero their secrets;
I'm sure they won't know where to start,
but without a shadow of a doubt,
the beauty in their heart sets them apart.

Strength hot like fire,
a spark of resilience and pride,
fuelled by the determination
to live the life that they decide.

Rising from the ashes
of every time they've been burnt,
each occasion they've been plagued by doubt
or punished for everything that they weren't.

A hero's superpower is their courage
to get up and step up to each new day.
Refusing to hide away from the world,
this isn't a game they're prepared to lose or
play.

*Standing a little taller
than they did the day before,
they protect themselves with the love they need
to end the battle and win the war.*

*A hero is amongst us.
A heart of gold gets them through.
Their identity is no longer lost;
the hero is you.*

When I was younger, I always wanted to have superpowers of flight and invisibility. After doing two skydives in my twenties, I would still choose flight in a heartbeat. (From experience, I would 100% recommend doing as high a jump as you can, should the urge take you and the opportunity arise. My body took longer to acclimatise after a 10,000ft drop than it did from a 16,500ft fall—and besides, the higher your ascent, the more time you have to enjoy the experience and take in the view on the way down.) However, I'm older now and age has given me perspective. Yes, I would still love to be able to fly, but I would choose other powers too. I would choose to be able to cure any disease or illness. I would want to be able to speak Italian fluently (I've been learning for what feels like a lifetime and I doubt I'll ever be as good as I want to be, so a little supernatural assistance would be gratefully appreciated). I would like to have perfect vision or to be able to avert disasters and end suffering. I don't think I'm asking for much. The pre-school children I work with would probably agree with me, to an extent, as obviously some of the best superheroes can fly as part of their daily lives and all round 'super-ness'. But they would likely also say 'shoot webs', 'be a rainbow unicorn', 'freeze everything' or 'blast to the moon'. My point is, as we grow up and our lives unfold, our priorities and perceptions change. Our hopes and dreams and fears and fantasies ebb, flow, and evolve along with us—sometimes for the better, sometimes for the worse. I guess it's only through lived experience that we realise what we're truly capable of, and which dreams, when brought to fruition, could actually destroy us.

During 2019, I achieved invisibility. Rather than it being miraculous, powerful or life-enhancing, it was degrading, agonising, and soul-destroying. It wasn't a gift from a supernatural realm, but an inconsistent and powerful response from an ex, who looked through me, past me, around me, and anywhere but at me, in the most public way possible. We worked together, and I lost count of the number of days I'd will myself out of my car on a morning to face whatever the day would bring. I dreaded catching sight of him, a stranger who had seen everything but who now saw nothing at all. I would often walk through the building, trying to catch a glimpse of my reflection or someone else's gaze. Not for egotistical purposes, but to prove to myself that I still existed, that I was still visible to someone, and I hadn't ceased to be seen by everyone—despite seemingly ceasing to matter to one. I honestly had moments where I thought I'd entered a parallel universe. I questioned whether, if I screamed loudly enough, I'd stand a chance of being heard or if my voice would disappear into a void, given that my body and presence had seemingly disappeared into invisibility and irrelevance. I felt utterly disposable. I eventually realised that others saw me, but my self-esteem was on the floor by that point, so I perceived that they saw me as inadequate and worthless. In an ironic and vicious circle, I felt more invisible with each passing day. Some days, he would see me and there would be a flicker of acknowledgment, as cold and waning as a dying ember on the flames of what had once been the most complicated relationship I've ever been in. Between that and being ignored, I honestly can't work out which killed me the most. I lost my mind and any desire to get out of bed in the morning. This will either come across as an extreme reaction to a relationship breakup, or painfully relatable. Although it was one of the most horrific chapters in my story so far, for multiple reasons, it wasn't the end of the story. I didn't scream into the abyss, run through the office naked or attempt to draw any attention to myself at all. Instead, I remembered myself and realised that I was here and that I had choices. The choices I'd made up to that point had been responsible for getting me there and the ones I made now would be responsible for getting me through, past, and beyond this. I realised I had to choose wisely. I had to choose my mental health and I had to choose myself; the two came hand-in-hand.

I was a mental health first-aider at work, and I reached out to one of my fellow first aiders—my colleague and my friend. Recognising the signs of my own imminent breakdown, I let my mask slip. My heart burst open and my pain came tumbling out in a sea of tears, words, pain, and confusion. Without judgement, without interruption or opinion or a metaphorical box of sticking plaster suggestions, she listened. She heard me, and she saw me. She reminded me that I was alive, my pain was real and justified, and I needed to give myself time to process and heal. The relationship had happened in an instant, but the aftermath was prolonged and painful, and I'm still processing it. I realised that I needed to take back some control of my life and my emotional reactions. I contacted a counselling service offered, ironically enough, through the health scheme at work, and I hoped that an external service affiliated with the place that was killing me would actually help save me. Once again, I found myself reaching out for that lifesaving lifeboat.

Counselling isn't for everyone. It doesn't have to come in the form of talking therapy or sharing your soul and secrets with a stranger, who you must inherently trust and gel with on some level for the sessions and the process to be of any benefit. It's not necessarily about visualisation and breathing techniques. It doesn't have to involve writing anything down, completing weekly tasks, and implementing tools to overcome something or bring about a physical or psychological change. Yes, all of those elements can be involved, and I've experienced them all to varying degrees over the years; it depends upon the type of counselling you choose and what you're trying to achieve. I've had talking therapy and CBT (cognitive behaviour therapy) over the years, and whilst some sessions and branches of therapy were more beneficial and comfortable than others, I learned something from all of them and I don't class any of it as wasted time or energy.

Therapy looks different for everyone. It could involve talking with a friend or a professional or both. Choose whoever makes you feel most at ease, the most seen, heard and validated, and who can offer you the safest space to tell your story, or whichever part you feel most comfortable sharing. The other person's role isn't to give you the answers or, as I'd previously hoped, to 'fix' you or the situation. Theirs is only one opinion, which you can consider, but you don't have to take as gospel. Personally, I now don't think it's healthy to look upon yourself as needing fixing, as you're not broken; however you may feel to the contrary. You're a whole person who needs to reconnect with and believe in yourself again—to heal, to reflect, to rebuild and to move forward in a new, more positive direction.

Some people find talking therapy groups helpful. There's an emphasis on creating a group dynamic, on sharing experiences and strategies, triumphs and pain, and reducing the sense of isolation and alienation. Groups can offer escapism and an emotional, physical, and creative outlet. Groups such as art classes, walking groups, bereavement and grief groups, and even groups that aren't established for the purpose of therapy, can all offer refuge and a chance to rebuild and repair. Consider activities that require you to be present in the moment, to be a part of a team or to explore a part of yourself other than that which is consuming you and causing you pain. For me, talking with someone professional and impartial helped immensely, as they weren't a girlfriend extolling my finer points, with a lot of love and a degree of bias. I was, however, eternally grateful for the therapy offered through friendship, too.

The last therapist I saw, across six talking therapy sessions, helped me come to a realisation that was borne out of an almost-irrelevant, passing comment. It felt so significant it stopped me in my tracks. The therapist observed that when we experience a positive moment, we want more of it. In that statement I heard 'addiction'. I realised with clarity that I was addicted to the intoxicating high of a good moment, whether that moment arises from time with friends, family or, perhaps more poignantly, within a relationship. I'd never realised how detrimental this path was until I was too far down it. I was addicted to love and being in a loving relationship—although I didn't know what that looked like in reality, as I've never been in one. Even exes who've said those all-important three words ultimately contradicted themselves through their actions; they invalidated them through their subsequent harmful words and hasty retreats. I've wanted it so badly that I've done enough loving, enough planning for the future, and enough fighting for the relationship for the both of us. When they walked away, I was left broken and empty. They invested so little in comparison that they could carry on, unscathed and unaware of the devastation they'd caused, which I subsequently lived through. And that's when the self-doubt became more real; I took their lack of care and love to be a reflection of me and not them. I saw myself through their eyes...as not attractive, loveable, interesting, good, etc, etc. enough to love, to commit to or to fight for. I came to believe it enough, so that it is exactly what I have portrayed.

Through therapy, a lot of soul-searching, from conversations with friends, and outpourings to my tear-stained reflection, I realised that allowing anyone from my past to take up such an active role in my present head space was slowly killing me. It was taking my sanity and destroying my chances of peace, happiness, and purpose—now and in the future. With each conscious mental trek down memory lane, each replaying of a conversation, a feeling or a lost moment in time, I was putting a metaphorical knife to a different part of my skin. With each tear shed, each mental recrimination, each 'what if' scenario revisited and reimagined, and each moment of complete emptiness and worthlessness that followed, I was drawing from a deeper reserve of blood and emotions. I was causing myself more pain, and the scars were getting more visible. The pain behind my eyes was either making me numb or leaving evidence of its story etched on my cheeks. I needed to step away from the knife drawer. I needed to leave the past where it belonged and take an active role in my present. I needed to make possible all the amazing tomorrows that I so desperately wanted and needed, and which have thankfully arrived since that moment in 2019.

I can't tell you what therapy or healing looks like for you. Through my own experience, I can tell you that no matter how strong your support network or inner resilience is, the process needs to start with you. It must start with you asking for help. It must start with you putting yourself first—every last physical and psychological piece of you—as you take steps towards a future you want and deserve. It starts with you realising and vocalising that you're enough, that you always have been enough, and that the present might be as scary as hell, but the future could be better than you can currently imagine. Recovering is not about burying your past, but finding the tools and support to make peace with it. It starts with you recognising the hero that you are, for all that you are, and letting your strength, potential, and dreams take flight.

Never pick a petal or two

I love me.
I love me not.
Pick a petal;
watch it rot.

Abraham Lincoln is attributed to the quote, 'There are no bad pictures; that's just how your face looks sometimes.'

This strikes a chord with me as I'm highly self-critical. Research data, and the views and experiences others have shared with me over the years, shows that I'm not alone. A House of Commons Committee report in August 2022 highlighted that 80% of their respondents agreed or strongly agreed that their mental health was detrimentally impacted by their body image. 61% agreed or strongly agreed that their body image had a negative impact upon their physical health. A Mental Health Foundation report in 2019 found that 19% of adults felt disgusted by their body image and 31% of teenagers felt ashamed because of the way they looked. Anxiety and depression stemming from a negative body image affected approximately 35% of teenage and adult respondents, with 13% experiencing suicidal thoughts as a result of their appearance. The same MHF report showed that 22% of adults and 40% of teenagers believed social media had a detrimental effect on how they viewed their own bodies.

Our faces are our identity. They're the first thing we tend to see when we look in a mirror, the first part of another person we focus on, and the thing we seem to judge the most harshly—as well as what we invest the most time and money into 'perfecting'. They are the canvas to every emotion we feel and every story we tell. They bear the visible signs that we've laughed, cried, lived, fought, lost, won, and aged. We conceal them behind masks of varying kinds. We inject time-defying lotions and potions into them. We pluck, pierce, decorate, and treat them in a seemingly endless pursuit to perfect and accept them. Yet, we're seemingly discouraged from ever fully embracing the unfiltered skin we're in. If I looked at myself in the mirror right now, if I'm being totally honest, my first instinctive response would likely be to notice my flaws... and I hate admitting to that level of self-deprecation. I'm not proud of this vanity, but it follows me like my shadow; a persistent stalker, most prominent in the cold light of day, whilst other insecurities take over the night shift. So, why am I telling you this, when my objective is supposed to be to inspire self-love, and to help you see the beauty in our human faces? Well, I want to be honest when I tell you that weakness accompanies strength. Silver linings are only possible when the sun hugs the clouds, and love is the light that permeates the shadows. The positive and the negative come hand in hand, each one the other's necessary foe, like conflicting conjoined twins.

I speak from experience. To give you some context around my struggle with my self-esteem and my problematic relationship with my reflection, it started when I was five. I had a face only a mother could love. It buckled under the weight of large, round-rimmed glasses—the sort that wouldn't have looked out of place on Deidre Barlow or the base of a jam jar. My hair was cut in a bowl-style, as if an actual bowl had been used to shape and sculpt it, although I'm assured this wasn't actually the case. At that age, I was just about cute enough to get away with it. Fast-forward seven years and picture the scene: I'm a 12-year-old Year 8 pupil, in a secondary school that was tantamount to a home for delinquents (just to clarify, I wasn't one of them. I was there through bad luck rather than merit). I was sat in the centre of the room in a history lesson, led by a female teacher who was young enough to know a little about sisterhood and how to honour it, yet on this occasion, she chose not to. The focus of the lesson was the Roundheads and Cavaliers. As she painted a verbal picture of the time and place, she decided a visual reference point was required, (evidently, an image on the whiteboard wouldn't have sufficed). She called on me to stand up, so she could better make her point about the Roundheads' appearance (who were infamous for cropping their hair close to their heads). If I'd been a metaphorical plant in that classroom, my teacher would not only have publicly plucked every petal from me in that one excruciatingly painful display of humiliation and social suicide, she would have also uprooted my entire body from its life source and cast me onto the compost heap. The fact that I can recall this event in graphic detail over 25 years later pays testament to how scarring her words and intentions were for me in that moment.

A few years later, I was subjected to the nickname Velma from Scooby-Doo (this time, by a fellow student, rather than someone paid to educate me), until I left school and finally discovered contact lenses and a decent, flattering hairstyle. Just to be clear, I have absolutely nothing against glasses. They suit a lot of people and I resent the fact that all 'geeks' in animations and films are seen sporting them as their trademark badge of social rejection. That is, until Hollywood comes along and turns them into a beauty queen or superhero, minus the 'bins'.

The reason I'm sharing these mortifying examples of how it took me almost two decades to learn to appreciate and accept my own reflection, is to reassure you that my words aren't hollow. They haven't been lifted from positive affirmations and self-love mantras, which can be as sweet as candyfloss, with just as little substance. I've lived through the names and negative connotations, the derogatory labels, the shame and self-pity. I know how necessary it is to be able to look at your reflection with pride and gratitude, and to give two metaphorical fingers to anyone who uses their words to hurt rather than to heal.

It's bullying, it's cruel, and it's small. It's devastating when it's done to us by others, especially those we're closest to, and who we're our most vulnerable with (I've been there, too). But it's unforgivable when society turns us upon ourselves and causes us to be the victim of our own bullying, to the point where we destroy ourselves from the inside out. Like a plant, we too are beautiful, unique, and as fragile as we're strong. We've spent a lifetime growing, withstanding the elements, fighting for survival, and another day above ground. Just as we discourage children from picking the petals from a plant and plucking it from the ground whilst it still blooms, we should resist the urge to pick ourselves apart. We destroy ourselves daily, with one negative comment, one 'If only I was...' and one detrimental act of seeking to improve what is already there and already enough, after another. We may each experience a complex relationship with our body, during and throughout our lifetime. A body that's both our greatest armour and the only place we'll ever permanently live. Yet, we go into battle against it with the war we wage upon ourselves. We destroy it with a daily diet of derogatory comments, whilst starving it of life-sustaining acceptance and gratitude.

My attitude towards my body now is one of gratitude. I've been short-sighted since starting school and I've accepted this as part of my identity. I have, in truth, always resented my imperfect eyesight, but in both 2012 and 2018, I nearly lost my sight, caused by an abrasion and ulcer to my cornea. It was so traumatic and terrifying, that I could potentially have lost the one thing I most valued yet took for granted, that when the consultant tried to take

Never pick a petal or two

a biopsy, I promptly passed out and came round on the lap of a male medic. I was in shock for weeks. I took daily visits to the hospital to have drops applied and the ulcer monitored. It was only by a stroke of luck that it had formed where it had. If it had been millimetres higher, it would have permanently affected my field of vision. I'm human, so I still find myself taking my imperfect sight for granted, but I'm also now consciously grateful for it every single day. I think we're all used to giving unconscious thought to something that has always been with us and which is a part of us, without question or threat. This is the attitude I have towards my body—I now view it with love and a deepening awareness of how fragile, impermanent, and incredible it is.

I don't know you or your health and circumstances, but as a broad piece of advice, I would encourage you to always see your body as the life-sustaining gift it is. I hope you come to recognise that the one part of your body you pay the least attention to, which you give the fewest compliments to or which you resent and bemoan the most, may be the part that someone else wishes they had.

Returning to the quote at the start of this chapter...maybe we could all challenge ourselves to be kinder to and about ourselves.

How many times do we occupy ourselves with the pursuit of getting the 'perfect, spontaneous selfie', only to filter, edit, and crop it before it can be shared publicly? I don't know about you, but I'm old enough to remember the days when we had no idea how a photo would turn out until we collected it from a processing stand. I remember desperately hoping that the majority of the limited prints I had per film would be in focus, without a finger obscuring the lens! In my opinion, the best photographs are those that capture natural, candid human moments: loving conversations, playfulness between friends, snapshots of wild abandon, and everything in-between. Instead of scrutinising the picture for flaws or everything that it isn't, I can't help feeling that we should appreciate it for everything that it is, i.e. the moment, the people, and the feelings it captures.

Rather than looking for perfection in a person, in yourself, in a moment or a photograph, revel in the moments and cherish the memories. You'll never get that moment back again; you'll never get another shot at taking that exact same shot or capturing that memory. When the moment has passed and the person has gone, that photo and those fading memories will be all you're left with and what you cling to. I'm certain that we would no longer care about perfection then; we'd just wish that we had that person and that time back again—whether that person is someone else or a version of us that's gone forever. Perhaps we all need to be kinder to ourselves and about ourselves, both in the moment and when those moments are a memory in our hands.

Remember the moment when you took the photograph. Who were you with? How did you feel about those people? How did you feel about yourself? What was happening in your life in that moment? Where were you, and what had it taken, physically or emotionally, to get you there? The answer to all these questions matters more than the final image. See a person's character shine through in their facial expressions, pose, and perhaps their inability to look at the correct part of the camera or smile naturally as the moment is captured. (Think of the infamous episode of Friends, where Chandler is perfectly able to smile as a genuine expression of happiness, until the moment a camera appears and he instead looks painfully and comically constipated). The bigger picture is often more important and meaningful than any of the individual elements that make up the image. In a world where we're increasingly encouraged to use filters as an 'enhancement', and to critique and condemn people for being authentically human, it's more critical than ever to be less critical. We need to remind ourselves that our beauty is evident and indisputable. The fact we're alive, that we're living, thriving, and surviving, to different degrees on any given day, is something to be proud of and grateful for. The only person we should ever compare ourselves to is the one we were yesterday.

Anxiety, depression, self-loathing, and body-shaming issues are real, unique, and painfully prevalent today—and at an increasingly young age. We need to break the toxic culture of labels, definitions, and personifications of beauty. We need to reject these societal stereotypes, before society and social media turn us against ourselves and we forget how to love the body that sustains us; the only one we'll ever have. We need to stop berating our bodies for looking and functioning the only way they know how. I understand that this is easier said than done, and I know there's no overnight fix to remedy a lifetime's worth of picking ourselves or being picked apart. I have friends who hate having their pictures taken in any situation and will physically remove themselves from the shot. They negatively compare themselves to others and use words about themselves that break my heart, as they cannot see the obvious beauty in themselves that others see in them. That beauty is visible, and it's much more than skin-deep.

When we use negative descriptions about ourselves, we're damaging ourselves—sometimes physically, and always emotionally and psychologically. If we allow these words to permeate our minds, infiltrate our self-talk, and cloud and distort our view of ourselves, the scars could last a lifetime and become our legacy. Imagine saying negative, confidence-eroding words to a child. The thought horrifies me, and yet we do this to our inner child daily…each time we turn away from them in disgust or shame or when we label them as anything less than enough. Each time you say anything negative, untrue or harmful to yourself or about yourself, you strip away a layer of protection—an essential part of your armour and identity. This is tantamount to plucking petals from a flower to remove its power, purpose, and beauty.

I'm not saying that establishing a loving relationship with yourself is easy, but it's absolutely necessary and it should be nurtured daily. It starts in our brain; we need to rewire the compulsion to be negative and harmful when we see and discuss ourselves. Rather than listening to that default critical voice that resides within us, and which makes itself known when we look at ourselves—in the flesh or retrospectively—we need to drown out that voice with a genuine compliment or sentiment of gratitude. Rather than looking at an aspect of your body that you dislike because it doesn't function perfectly, try considering how much more problematic your daily life would be if it wasn't there or if it didn't function at all. This may sound too easy, and honestly, it takes practice, persistence, and patience, but it can make a world of difference. What a difference it might make if we were able to look at the silver lining, however faint it might be, rather than the cloud, which we perceive to be overwhelming and oppressive.

If there's a part of yourself that you don't like cosmetically, is there anything non-invasive you can do to change it? Or could you accentuate another feature instead that you do like, which will give you a positive aspect to focus on?

There's so much we can say about kindness, but the quote, **'In a world where you can be anything, be kind'** seems particularly relevant and underrated. Beauty shines through from within, in the form of the words we speak, the

Never pick a petal or two

love we share, the impact we have, the time we give, and the legacy we leave. It breaks through whatever perceived 'cracks' we have, in the form of wrinkles, imperfections and human fallibility. If beauty really is in the eye of the beholder, let us practise looking upon ourselves with respect, love, and gratitude, and with our eyes clear and wide open. The road to self-love won't be easy, but it's one we need to take and which we need to teach our children how to navigate, through our example.

Several years ago, I came across the 'sand flea experiment', which I think provides a deeply profound and disturbing insight into human behaviour, when we consider people in place of fleas. Let me explain. Fleas are known for their ability to jump to considerable heights, and here our first flea-to-human comparisons can be drawn. Scientists decided to observe, manipulate, and monitor this behaviour. They placed a number of fleas in a glass jar. Immediately, the fleas relied upon their innate instincts and they jumped out. This led the scientists to introduce a lid, to seal the fleas within the jar. In that moment, the lid became the physical and metaphorical glass ceiling to these test fleas and, crucially, their future offspring.

The scientists noticed that the fleas

continued to jump, but now, only as high as the lid—which was all their barrier to the outside world would allow. Soon enough, their behaviour altered so that they jumped to just below the lid, meaning that they never physically reached it. Their imposed restrictive surroundings conditioned their behaviour in the way they interacted with and inhabited their environment. Ultimately, once the jar and its lid were both permanently removed, the fleas retained the memory and psychological imprint of their physical limitations and they never again jumped higher than the lid had previously allowed. What I found even more fascinating was in the scientists' further studies, once those fleas reproduced, their offspring failed to jump any higher than their parents had been conditioned to jump. The experiment had effectively, and perhaps unwittingly, created an intergenerational group of fleas who behaved in exactly the same way for the rest of their lives; never jumping beyond their perceived barriers or challenging their conditioned behaviour.

Do you see where I'm going with this analogy? Have you ever considered how our words can detrimentally define, imprison, and destroy us over a consistent and continuous period of time? Our self-talk is the most

Never pick a petal or two

powerful tool and weapon we have at our disposal, and we use it against ourselves on a daily basis. It's the voice that never leaves us and the one we can either choose to ignore or succumb to. I've already mentioned the importance of speaking to ourselves with love, with regards to our physical appearance, and learning to compliment what we've spent years making excuses for and criticising about ourselves. When we label ourselves negatively and let our inner voice limit or decide our potential, self-worth, and aspirations, we poison ourselves from within. That kind of damage can last a lifetime and become lethal. Each time you tell yourself something derogatory or untrue, you're not only preventing yourself from succeeding, but often, from trying at all. Your relationship with yourself bleeds into and infects every external relationship you have. How you see yourself informs others of the level of worth you place upon yourself, and what you expect and will accept in return.

Your worth is limitless, and I don't need to have met you personally to know that. To reiterate a point I made in the chapter titled 'The miracle is you': you're miraculous and you are enough. We live in a world that feels increasingly cold, emotionless, and lacking in meaningful and nurturing interactions. So, let the deepest, most real and loving relationship be the one you have with yourself. Nurture yourself from within. Polish your petals, rather than pluck at them with scorn, shame or self-deprecation, however much jest your comments are veiled in.

How many times have you received a compliment only to bat it away dismissively and uncomfortably, through fear of not knowing what to do with it?

Compliment: 'I like your hair.' **Deflection**: 'Oh, I washed it for once.'

Compliment: 'You did great today, your presentation was fantastic.' **Deflection**: 'I'm just doing my job and it could definitely have gone better. I lost my place halfway through, did you not notice?'

Compliment: 'You look beautiful.' **Deflection**: 'Who, me? Hardly!'

Compliment: 'I love you.' **Deflection**: 'You have to say that, you're my friend/sister/husband/wife. You're biased.'

I don't know if any of these exchanges sound remotely familiar, but I'm sure we've all deflected a compliment without acknowledging or appreciating it. I honestly have no idea why this has become our automatic and destructive default. The greatest thing we can do for ourselves, learn for ourselves, and teach others, is to love ourselves exactly as we are. We must actively silence that critical inner voice and celebrate all that we are, rather than anything we're not. If we were to actively take note of the negative self-talk we endured during an average day, we would no doubt have several scars to punctuate the narrative. The adage 'sticks and stones may break my bones, but words will never hurt me' is the epitome of irony and deception. You are human, and by that very definition and your very existence, you're fallible and imperfect. You have the potential to make mistakes and have many 'first attempts in learning' moments. Recognise these as your springboard, not your jar lid or glass ceiling. Once you routinely recognise and remind yourself of this, your relationship with yourself will hopefully flourish and set the standard for how you demand and deserve to be treated by others. Nurture, rather than pick, each of your individual petals, so that others will be encouraged to do the same.

Action point for kindness and lasting change:

Try giving yourself a genuine compliment every day.

It could be something physical, such as

A Glass Glued with Gold

telling yourself that the colour you're wearing suits you; that your skin looks healthy; that your hair is co-operating, or your new make-up is worth the money. It could even be as simple as telling yourself that you look better, healthier, less tired or happier than you did the day before.

It might be character driven. Maybe the way you dealt with a stressful situation, a challenge you overcame, a positive effect you had on someone else or a difference you were able to make. It could perhaps be reminding yourself that you are good, clever, capable, and beautiful (etc.) enough.

As you think of these compliments and positive attributes, write them down. It's up to you where you put them. Consider somewhere visible, such as post-it notes on your bedroom mirror, inside your car's sun-visor or dotted around your house, depending on the people you live with. Perhaps you could conceal them somewhere more private, such as within your purse, a notebook or your phone; whatever feels right and most beneficial for you. Wherever you put them, make them accessible, so you can read and re-read them as often as you need to.

Why not extend the love outwards and start a new family tradition, by leaving complimentary notes for your loved ones to find? Imagine what a difference it could make to the start of your day if you found a compliment on the kettle, a note of encouragement on the bathroom door or a token of love or appreciation within your cereal box.

(I'm not being naive here. I'm not suggesting you get up at 5am every day to set up a paper trail of love notes for yourself and anyone else you might live with. But random, spontaneous, and heartfelt words and acts of kindness, positivity, and appreciation can change a person's day, outlook or relationship with themselves.)

It isn't an exaggeration to say that making a person feel seen, heard, and valued has the potential to save a life. That could be a person in your life or the person in the mirror. No one ever truly knows what another person is dealing with behind their mask or beneath the surface. Maybe, over time, that saved life could be your own.

Use your words as your strength and your protection, to glow through what you go through in life. Life can be difficult enough, without going to war with yourself.

Do you want to live this way?

Non piangere perché una cosa finisce, sorridi perché é accaduta
(Don't cry because it's over, smile because it happened)

I didn't see the curtain fall,
but it took my breath away
and my heart along with it,
plummeting excruciatingly
as I bite the bullet
and swallow the pill.
I choke on the bitterness
and denial
over the realisation
that this is the hand that fate has dealt.
I find myself in the pool of my grief,
drowning in the sudden senselessness
of shock and abandonment
that is mine to bear,
borne from a choice I did not make,
but it became my narrative.
I love you, but that is not enough
to disarm the truth,
too unbearable to stomach,
yet it repeats on me
with each breath,
each blink,
each memory that spills from my eyes,
the invisible map of my grief,

etched along my cheek
which I navigate alone
as you are gone.
And that truth breaks my heart.
I catch my breath,
suffocating on the silence,
which stifles my words
that try to escape,
but linger instead, unspoken and unheard.
I have never felt more alone.
So I hold myself up
and I hold my nerve
as I hold you
for a final time.
But all the time in the world
will never be enough.

I wonder if knowing
ever cushions the blow,
as the bruising and the scars
are inevitable and permanent,
regardless of whether they're viewed
through the eyes of foresight or hindsight.
I don't want to sound petulant,
but I silently scream into the void
you left in your wake;
this isn't fair and I wish
I didn't have to miss you
as much as I always will.

I don't know about you, but I really struggle to let go of things in life. I'll rephrase that—it's less things and more people that my heart clings onto. I hate saying goodbye.

Missing someone comes cloaked in darkness, leaving an emptiness that gnaws away at you until you feel hollow, nostalgic, and possibly resentful. I think this Italian translation of Dr. Seuss's adage is beautiful in its simplicity, even if it might seem unachievable or fanciful in the initial period of separation or for as long as that separation might last. Don't get me wrong, not every ending should be mourned and not every person you lose is a loss. Some goodbyes are most definitely a blessing in some degree of disguise. But for those goodbyes that cause genuine heartbreak and whose effects are devastating, how do you deal with it without letting it consume you? How do you ultimately achieve a level of acceptance and closure?

To be clear, I'm not specifically or exclusively talking about missing a partner after a break-up. I think that sentiment of 'smiling because it happened' can only apply if you both mutually agreed to end the relationship; if you parted as friends or if the end didn't come as some brutal and bruising bolt out of the blue. Enough time needs to have passed for the smile to be borne from genuine nostalgic gratitude, rather than being painted on in a pained portrayal of strength and indifference. This rhetoric is a comfort to me because it offers a perspective of calm contemplation. You can't control who enters or leaves your life, at what point or how long they will stay. You can't predict the impact they will have, the way in which they'll change you, and the footprints they'll leave behind on your heart or your mind. But you can control how you respond to their absence and how you cope with the space they leave in your life, mind, and heart in the wake of their departure.

Sometimes, the way we choose or are able to respond to a situation is the only autonomy we have. That could be our only source of power over the narrative. I wrote the poem at the start of this chapter with all kinds of loss in mind and considering the grief that every final goodbye is shrouded in, whether derived from death or desertion. Maybe it will resonate with you on some level, if you've ever suffered the brutality of saying goodbye against your will. I think what I struggle with the most is the lack of control you have over the impact that anyone else—their presence, their actions, their words and their departure—will have on your life. Yes, you hold the pen. You're responsible for writing your own story and you can rename any life event as a 'plot twist' at any point, however far it deviates from the original plan. Yet it's far harder to predict the level of pleasure or pain any character will bring to your story, how meaningful or memorable they will become, and how much they may ultimately change everything. You don't always get to plan the ending. But you must participate and ultimately live through it, long after the relationship or the person has died or their presence in your life has faded. You survived, and that's your poisoned chalice.

You are already made of gold. Now you need to use what you have to seal the cracks between each shattered piece of the you that you thought you knew before. Let it shine through the perfect imperfections of the you that's left behind. However clichéd and romanticised that might sound, trust me, you can do it. The fact you're still here means you're already making significant progress on that journey. At no point will it be easy. In fact, it will likely be one of the most unbearable things you will ever do. But their decision is not a death or even a life sentence for you; it's just the end of that part of your life. As I touched upon in an earlier chapter, time brings about many things. In the aftermath of loss, time may bring about an adjustment, a strength, a gratitude or a state of healing—if you're patient enough to meet and accept it when it arrives.

Not everyone will play the role you expected or wanted them to. Not everyone will be in it for the long haul. People will let you down. People will leave. People will love you, but not in the way you wanted or needed, not in the way you loved them, not enough or not at all. People's life choices will take them on different paths, and your paths may never cross again, despite your promises and best intentions. Even though you might not realise it at the time, some goodbyes are forever. Some goodbyes are said so naturally, with the assumption that there will always be more. Each one takes its place as naturally as one breath following another, until one, unsuspectingly, becomes the last. Or alternatively, you know before you say it that this will be the goodbye that punctuates your story with a definitive ending, and there won't be a sequel. In all honesty, I don't know which is more brutal.

Several years ago, I had a colleague who became the type of friend everyone needs in their life. He could read me like a book, and he made the effort to hear the unspoken words just as much as those I said aloud. We could talk about anything and everything, no limitations, no judgements. At a point in my life when I felt invisible, he saw me, and I'm forever grateful to him for that. I lost him to a different hemisphere and time zone, and I knew that last goodbye would possibly be the last time I saw him. We've kept in touch since, but I really miss the person I saw every day, the person who made me laugh and believed in me, and who was a genuinely good and utterly unique egg. That was a different loss to navigate my way through—how do you miss someone who hasn't died or hurt or left you, they've just left the country? Relationships, both romantic and platonic, are as complex and fragile as they are beautiful. Each time you open yourself up to loving someone, caring about them, becoming emotionally invested in their life, and committing to being there through their highs and lows, you accept the risk that silently skips along with the reward. The risk of them leaving, the risk of one of you hurting the other, of one person being more invested in your relationship than the other, or the risk of life events outside your control upending the status quo. There's always the risk that one conversation, one life choice or one moment in time has the potential to change everything.

Unlike romantic relationships, I think friendships evolve more naturally. There are fewer expectations, and less need to label and define yourselves as friends or to calculate the success or longevity of your friendship. Have you ever had the conversation with a friend along the lines of, 'So, what exactly are we doing here? Would you like to be my friend?' Or, to quote 50 Cent, 'I'll be your best friend, if you promise you'll be mine.' No? Me neither. Yet I've trodden this road countless times whilst embarking on a new romantic relationship, wanting to the point of needing that label, that definition, that reassurance. Society has perpetuated the belief that a label, an anniversary date or a definitive moment, such as becoming 'Insta-official' (back in the day it used to be Facebook-official, how early 2000s that feels now!), somehow seals your fate as safe and shatterproof against any kind of pain or ending. Crazy is as crazy does, I guess.

There's a risk of loss or loneliness in any relationship. It can hurt like hell, but it's worth the pain, and you can always return from hell. But surely, to never try due to the fear of goodbyes, or to live your life bearing the scars of past losses that you could have never predicted or prevented, well, that's got to be a living hell of its own.

Goodbyes may be painful and unexpected, and they can totally blindside you. We can all become overly emotionally invested and spend too long looking back at a time that no longer exists. But I believe that is the double edge to the sword, and I guess it's what makes us appreciate each new memory we're allowed to make, as nothing is guaranteed.

Please don't allow a person to determine your happiness or a relationship to consume you. Be committed to the person you're with, the moment you're in, and the future you hope to build. But please don't sideline or sabotage yourself within this scene. If the curtain falls to a crescendo of suffocating silence and abandonment, your pursuit of starting over will depend upon your ability to see your new path. Use your enoughness to guide you forward along it. Exist in conjunction with, not in the shadows of, anyone else. They will then only ever be able to enhance your light with their presence rather than extinguish it with their absence.

Goodbyes will come, but experience has taught me that you can armour yourself against some of the pain by aiming to leave each person happier, more loved, and more assured than you found them. Treat each meeting as if it could be your last. Whilst we're told that we only have one chance to make a first impression on another person, we perhaps forget that every meeting with them could potentially be the last, without any forewarning. Handle each encounter with care, gratitude, and love, as we also only have one chance to make a last impression. Hindsight can come with regrets and a replay, but never a rewind.

If you see something beautiful in someone—whether that's someone in your life or someone in the mirror—tell them. Give that genuine compliment. Tell them you're proud of them and explain why. Share laughter like it's oxygen. If you're both tactile people, hug them as though you have all the time in the world, and that the only place in the world you want to be is right there, in that embrace, in that moment. Don't leave anything unsaid. This might all sound painfully obvious, but too many times I've walked away from a situation wishing I'd said more, wishing I could have appreciated it more, felt more, been more present, and been more honest. My yearning for a time machine is underpinned by a plethora of regrets. We say 'see you later' as if it's a given. But we're not privileged enough to be able to see beyond the here and now, and that illustrious 'later' may, in fact, never come.

'Friends come and go, like waves of the ocean, but the true ones stick, like an octopus on your face!'

Non piangere perché una cosa finisce, sorridi perché é accaduta

I love this quote. It may not be eloquent, realistic or poetically deep, but I feel it packs a powerful punch. Notice the octopus (or octopi) in your life; cling stubbornly onto every one of them in return, like a barnacle to a rock. For the people who entered your life on a temporary basis and didn't stay as long as you wanted or imagined they would, save a space for them in your heart until a time when they may return. Otherwise, wish them well and rise above anything you may have felt in the aftermath of their goodbye. Not every partner will be your lobster (yes, I am quoting Friends!) and not every friend will be your octopus, but each one will have their place and purpose. Notice those whose arrival rode on the crest of a goodbye, when you lost an ex and gained a best friend, or when you left a job and a colleague became a lifelong friend. Maybe you'll realise that neighbours who moved away were really friends who once shared a postcode. Healing and beauty can come from a goodbye that once felt hurtful and ugly, and new chapters can follow old ones.

Like I said, I hate saying goodbye. Children I've taught, people I've loved, people who have inspired, changed, and accepted me, and people who I've simply wanted more time with, have all taken a space in my heart. Saying goodbye to each one was so difficult. Yet, for everything a goodbye can take from us, it can also give us memories, perspective, gratitude, and strength. A goodbye is only painful or significant when love is present. The pain of missing someone, and the appreciation for their existence and role in our lives, is only made possible by the presence of love. What is grief, other than a love that stubbornly refuses to die? Letting go of a person is uncomfortable, but sometimes, clinging onto what has passed can be excruciating. Don't lose yourself whilst trying to grieve the passing of time. Be present within each moment and take the memories forward with you—the good and the bad—as an honest memento of a life lived, shared, and impacted.

To experience a life before death, we must make ourselves vulnerable to all that life offers. This vulnerability becomes our strengthening armour. Love overcomes vast emptiness. It guides us through the unprecedented and the unpredictable, and the void where only time can help us make sense of the changes we've lived through. Love is our reason to move on, to carry on and to cling on—to the people, the life, and the hope left behind. That love comes from within. It comes from the deepest reserves of our hearts and minds...from our friendship groups, from our support systems, and our instinctive desire for survival. Not knowing what we may be walking into, who we may be walking away from, or where our journey will take us, can be paralysing. But it may also be the calming perspective that walks silently alongside us. It offers the reminder that a goodbye is only painfully possible because an initial hello once paved the way for its arrival, with a host of memories bridging the gap between one and the other.

Enough is enough

In the dark
at the end of the day,
your tears tell the story
of your bravery and pain,
which etches its narrative
down your cheek,
with ebbs and flows
and a rasping punctuation
of a defiant semi-colon
refusing to be silenced
in the wake of the fat lady's lament,
but rather, catches its breath
for an encore.
Although you may question
how many more straws
your back can take
as you contemplate
the reflection of the camel
or the ass before you.

You cast your mind back to a time
when it all made sense,
but it falters in the bowels of time
and you blink away the memories.
Blink and you miss it.
Blink and it's gone.
Your eyes promise persistence

above perfection
in a silent pact made to your ears
to allay the fears
of your heart,
which has heard it all before,
yet still chooses to believe
that tomorrow will be a better day,
because you are as you
as you have ever been
and that is your armour
and that is your strength
and that is the noose
they will attempt to hang you by,
if you give them enough.
Don't allow your reflections
to muddy the waters
or hold your heart hostage
in exchange for the essence of all that you are.
Instead, rise with each reverberation
of the whispered truth.

Enough is enough.

You are enough.
You are enough.
You are enough.

What does the word 'enough' mean to you? It's typically quantifiable in nature, in its use and purpose. 'Enough' often accompanies other subjective and invisible friends, such as *satisfactory, sufficient* and *adequate*. It can be shroud in favourable or judgemental connotations; to be described as any of the above is surely to be damned by the faintest of praise. But it can also hide in plain sight, appearing elusive, contradictory, and as fluid as sand running through our fingers.

Let's take these three examples:

A young child autonomously decides when they've had enough of a chosen activity, before their attention wanders and wanes and they move on to something new.

A parent will stringently decide when a child has had enough of their daily sugar consumption and removes temptation from sight and reach when that point arrives.

Our body instinctively decides when we've had enough sleep and wakes us up—unless an alarm clock, child, snoring partner or any other external factor gets there first.

In these cases, 'enoughness' seems to be a moment in time that's open more to interpretation than negotiation. It may result in conflict or frustration or, at the very least, a differing of opinion. Does your partner get to decide if you have enough pairs of shoes? Are we physically strong enough to independently carry that shopping or move that furniture? How readily will your child accept that you don't have enough money to buy the ice cream they want or enough time to read one more bedtime story? We each have the same number of hours in a day, but some of us feel that they're just not enough. In this case, we can be forever chasing more, like elusive pots of gold or our metaphorical tails, in order to be deemed productive or successful enough.

When 'enoughness' is visible and concrete, it's an easier concept to measure, to accept, and to comprehend. We can see whether the food we have will be enough to feed the people waiting to be served. We can visualise if there's enough water in the kettle or cutlery on the table. These things make sense to us from a very early age of living in and accepting the world, our perception of it, and our place within it. This is evidenced when a child decides that there's enough sand to fill their bucket, enough pieces to complete their jigsaw puzzle or enough teddies for everyone to have one each at the picnic. In my opinion, it's when 'enoughness' becomes a matter of opinion that it becomes a divisive, double-edged sword. Do you want it enough to fight for it? How hard should you fight or how long should you be willing to fight for? Do you care enough—about them or about yourself? Did you spend enough money on their anniversary or birthday present to demonstrate sufficient levels of love and thoughtfulness? Do you see them often enough? Do you spend enough time with yourself? Do you love them enough? Do they love you enough? It takes the consent, participation, and willingness of two people to begin and sustain a relationship—platonic or otherwise. Yet it can end on the decision of just one person, who decides that the love and motivation is not enough, on their part or yours. When this happens, even 'too much' love, effort or desire becomes less than enough to save it.

I personally believe that we should each be given the privilege to decide our own interpretation and definition of what enough looks and feels like in our relationships, in our lives, and in our mindsets. It's a word used as innocently as any other, and yet, dependent upon the context, it can be as loaded as ammunition. It can take a lifetime to form a healthy relationship with it, to a point where we trust it enough not to break our spirit, heart or defences.

My own relationship with being enough is a daily work in progress. Whilst I can now say that I weigh out the levels of my 'enoughness' against my own barometer more than I used to, I still find myself mentally handing over that decision to others from time to time. They will either erode, elevate or misalign my fragile scales, knowingly or otherwise. I have a feeling I'm not alone in managing this definition of what it means to be human and enough–day in, day out, dependent upon all the factors within and around me at any given moment.

Can you ask yourself in all honesty, is 'enough' a negative or positive concept for you? We bemoan, 'that's enough', 'enough is enough', and 'I've had enough'. These are often accompanied by echoes of frustration, desperation or despair. If you're told 'you are enough', on which side of the coin does that statement land for you: as a compliment or a condemnation? If it's the latter, how do we retrain our brains to flip the switch and reinterpret and reimagine the narrative?

What you go through doesn't define you. What you live through is a sentence in your life story, rather than a life sentence. The stones people throw at you are often self-directed, but as you get in their way, you bear the scars of the insecurities or ignorance of people who know better and need to do better. That's not your fault or your fate. You're brave in the face of cruelty, rejection, disappointment, and challenges. You choose to fight for another chance to rewrite your story, to have your voice heard, your heart fulfilled, and your potential realised; to make a difference and to matter. You've been resilient and determined enough to make that happen every day so far, and you can be again today. You're already enough of all you need to be in order to succeed.

You are brave enough.

You matter enough.

You're kind enough.

You are loved enough.

You're capable enough.

You're enough of all the things life has chipped away at. All the things you doubt, that you conceal and apologise for.

You're good enough to live the life you imagine. You're worthy enough to set your standards and expectations at heights others may have attempted to reduce, belittle or break.

Often, the greatest challenge is not achieving 'enoughness', but opening your eyes wide enough to look inwards and recognise that it's already there in abundance. Please hear me when I tell you that the existence or level of your enoughness does not depend upon any external validation.

Daily life, relationships, work pressures, unexpected conversations or confrontations;

the briefest moments in time can knock us all off kilter without a moment's notice.

It can cause us to question: *Did I control my emotions well enough as my child was struggling to control theirs?*
Was I prepared enough for that work situation?
Did I accept that apology sincerely enough?
Did I stand up for myself enough as I was being brought down?
Was I helpful or kind enough to the person who was struggling?
Was I brave enough to apologise for being wrong?

All of these questions are entirely natural. They are what enable us to nurture the seed of 'enoughness', and to reflect upon and enhance what we already carry. We all have the potential to be 'more'. That's what drives us to improve and develop. But we should see this as our driving force to move from one day to the next, rather than as a stick to beat ourselves with.

I've been trying to learn Italian for what feels like a lifetime. There has been progress and there's a level of skill there, but am I skilled enough to have a fluent conversation with a native Italian? No, frustratingly, I'm not...yet. But I want it enough and I'm capable enough, and my Italian mastery is as much of a work in progress as I am. I see it as my motivation, not my failing. Am I as intelligent and knowledgeable as I want to be or as I feel I ought to be, given my four decades of life experience, qualifications, and profession? Again, that would be a resounding no. But I reassure myself that I'm determined enough to use every day to try to fill where I'm lacking and to never stop learning and trying. I'm capable enough to be a better version of myself every day and that's my motivation. Yes, the word enough may be weighted with expectations, measurements, and consequences, but I personally believe that the way we learn to carry it determines both our relationship with it and the person in the mirror.

I hope your life is filled with enough shade to accentuate the light, and enough light to guide you through the dark. I hope that whomever you see in the mirror, for you alone, they are enough today, a little more than they were yesterday, and for the duration of all your unpromised tomorrows.

Tape and glue and cracks of gold

At points throughout life, as you navigate the emotional, physical, and psychological challenges of being human, you may feel any number of negative emotions. Please don't ever give those emotions or labels the power or permission to define you. You get a choice in how you put your pieces back together. Seal and solidify the cracks in the foundations of your life and your emotional armour with gold, so that they become a thing of beauty, value, and pride. They are a tattoo of your resilience and proof that you continue to survive.

We can spend a lifetime trying to have the time of our lives. We search for rainbows in storms, puddles to dance in, stars to guide us through the darkness, and silver linings to make the clouds less threatening.

Detailed below are just a small selection of insights and lessons I've discovered over the years, often when I've felt at my lowest. It's through these quotes, strategies, and escapisms that I've felt stronger, more empowered, and more able to look upon myself and my life with a little bit of pride. They represent some of the glue that gets me through. My hope is that they may, in some small way, be tools that you can use too. I hope they help you find the gold within you to repair whatever has happened to you—until you can say: *I want to live this way.*

- ♥ Your worth isn't defined by anyone else's ability, or lack of, to see and acknowledge it. Own it and don't offer any discounts to anyone, ever.

- ♥ Feed your mind, body, and soul, routinely and respectfully—especially when you're feeling starved of purpose and affection. This is when you need nurturing the most. You're basically a plant, just with more complex emotions. Get enough sunlight, water, vitamins, and rest.

- ♥ Not everyone will like, embrace or 'get' you...and that's okay. No one says they have to, and the world will continue to journey around the sun regardless of their opinion. For every person who isn't in your corner or on your wavelength, there are many more who will be.

- ♥ Try to create a sensory survival kit of:
- music you can listen to
- films you can watch
- words you can read

Tape and glue and cracks of gold

- food you can savour
- clothes you like to wear
- a person or item you like to hold close
- a person you can talk to, honestly and authentically
- a place you can mentally lose yourself in. Your own 'happy place', which evokes the positive and healing emotions and sensations you need to experience in that moment

(I can personally recommend the song '*I Am*' by Elaine Kristal, as a hauntingly soulful compilation of positive affirmations and reminders of our inherent human worth. Also, reading 'The Boy, the Mole, the Fox and the Horse', by Charlie Mackesy, is a beautiful, penetrative form of therapy, hope and love.)

The contents of your survival kit may change to meet whatever needs you have, but whomever and whatever is within it, make it personal, purposeful, and powerfully yours.

- ♥ If it isn't your fault, don't offer an apology to punctuate the silence, to settle an argument, to shoulder the blame or go to the trouble on someone else's behalf.

- ♥ Never compare yourself to anyone else. You

only see what they let you see, and 'perfection' may only last as long as it takes for the photograph to be taken or for a perception to be mistakenly planted in your mind. Rose is a deceptive tint and green is a destructive shade of anyone else's reality. For everyone you look at in envy, there is likely to be at least one person looking at you in the same way, which you may never even realise. You are not them, and that's more than okay. You are you, and what you bring to the table is totally unique and always more than enough.

♥ Collect your best memories, your moments of pride, your written or spoken notes of love, gratitude, and appreciation. Bury them deep within yourself. Let them feed your soul during any darker hours or days ahead. Let your own capabilities, achievements, and unique contributions sustain you when you're faced with a diet of despair and you're hungry for a sense of worth or meaning.

♥ If you can think of more reasons why you should do something than why you shouldn't, do everything you can to make it happen, until there's nothing more you can do. If it's meant to be a part of your story, do all that you can to allow and enable it.

- Be gentle with yourself. You're doing the best you can.

- Speak to yourself with kindness and look at yourself with love. Some days and moments will be harder than others, but you're more than capable of overcoming them. If you can be a good friend to others, your best friend should always be yourself. Otherwise, all other friendships are replacements, rather than enhancements, to the most important relationship of all...the one you have with yourself.

- Never allow anyone else to rewrite your history. Never hand over the pen to allow them to put words in your mouth or decide the level of pain you felt, how hurt you are entitled to feel or how long your grief should last. They do not get to decide what your healing should look like, what your happiness should look like, who you are as a result, or who you're capable of becoming. They might have heard your stories, but it's your heart alone that has experienced your pain.

- 💛 Find the glue that works for you. It could be:
- lie-ins
- exercise
- long soaks in the bath
- walking in nature
- being present during a sunrise
- being reflective during a sunset
- singing alone or collectively
- something that challenges and excites you
- a creative project
- a new hobby to start or an old hobby to revisit
- a group to join
- a skill to practise and enhance

It might be losing yourself in a box set or a book for the first time or the umpteenth time.

It could see you going for a drive with nowhere in mind, no time constraints, and your favourite playlist.

It could be a creative or mindful act that forces you to be present within the present as you create, appreciate or capture something uniquely personal.

It may be making memories with people you love, whilst talking about all the big and little things with the person or people you trust the most.

It may be losing yourself in an embrace or an act of physical or emotional intimacy.

Find your glue and use it with pride and enthusiasm, and without any apology.

- Fall forward.

- Find your tribe. This represents the people who know and love you for exactly who you are. They know and respect what you believe in, what you're prepared to accept and tolerate, what your dreams and aspirations are, and what you've been through to get to this point. They don't have to have been on the journey with you from the start. It doesn't matter when they entered your life. If:
  - they invest their time in you
  - their actions match their words
  - their belief in you matches or exceeds your belief in yourself
  - they celebrate your successes
  - they call you their family and, through time, they become yours
  - they saw you at your worst but never remind you of it

...these are your people and you deserve their friendship, their love, and all they have to give.

- As much as possible, try to add things to your memory bank rather than your to-do list.

- In life, don't allow anyone to put you in a box. Don't let anyone else define you as a person, limit or control your worth or your aspirations, or make you small to fit their own shortcomings. There's enough time in death to be contained.

- Don't be afraid to lose people along the way. It can be one of the most painful realisations to know that a person is harming you. Recognise when a relationship has become toxic or you're losing yourself in order to do what you've always done and be where you've always been. It can be the most prolonged and painful experience to walk away, but I promise you that you'll thank yourself when you do. You deserve better and you are worth more. Be brave in order to be free.

- Prioritise your mental health. It's not selfish or indulgent to do so; it's necessary, and the best investment you'll ever make.

- The bravest thing you can ever do is refuse

Tape and glue and cracks of gold

to accept defeat or become defined by a situation. Asking for help is <u>never</u> a weakness; it's the kindest and most proactive and positive thing you will ever do for yourself. It's not raising a white flag; it's the refusal to surrender.

- ♥ Experience as many elements of a 'GREAT DREAM' as possible, consistently and unapologetically. 'Action for Happiness' recommend incorporating ten positive and mindful activities into your daily interactions and experiences in order to live a more holistically healthy life:

Giving – Do things for others
Relating – Connect with people
Exercising – Take care of your body
Awareness – Live life mindfully
Trying out – Keep learning new things

Direction – Have goals to look forward to
Resilience – Find ways to bounce back
Emotions – Look for what's good
Acceptance – Be comfortable with who you are
Meaning – Be part of something bigger than yourself

- ♥ Never be afraid to take a risk, to step

outside of your comfort zone, to challenge your limits or ask yourself, 'Why not? What's the worst that can happen? What would I encourage a friend to do in the same situation? Do I want, need or deserve to live this way?'

- Start every day with the best intentions and a full heart. Accept yourself for your limitations and be proud of yourself for your strengths. End your day with gratitude for all that you are and all that you've experienced, enjoyed, and overcome. Forgive yourself for all that you're not. Applaud yourself for everything you've overcome to be at this point. You're still standing, still living, and still moving forward.

- Be in the moment. It's not about meditating with your eyes closed, nor regulating your breathing and visualising colours transcending through your body. It's about giving your undivided attention to the people you're with or the person in the mirror. It's about allowing yourself the chance to appreciate the smallest of sensations, rather than focusing solely on the end result. It's about the act of learning rather than the lesson itself. It's allowing the tears to fall. It's the warmth and depth of a hug, the fleeting yet lasting beauty of a sunset, a conversation with someone you love, and laughing with a child. It's feeling the pleasure in something temporary—like chocolate melting in your mouth, a hand in yours, the sincerity of a compliment, and the sound of silence amongst the chaos. It's the joy that happens whilst you're searching for happiness.

- Find pleasure in the smallest of things. Those that take up the most room in your heart and which are impossible to forget.

- Forgive yourself for it all.

- Be proud of yourself for every achievement —however big or small. Especially the small ones, because they're often huge.

- Love yourself before, and more than, you expect anyone else to. Otherwise, they'll never be able to love you enough, as your love for yourself will always be missing. Without that foundation, everything else will be built upon a fault line.

- 'A woman without a man is like a fish without a bicycle.' – A quote attributed to 'The Sydney Morning Herald' in 1975. I'm just saying...think about it.

- Step outside your comfort zone as often as you can. Your brain will fight you on it initially, but your heart and future self will thank you for it. It might just be the bravest, most life-affirming, and character-enhancing thing you ever do for yourself.

- If you can, do something by yourself, for yourself, as often as possible. A holiday or a weekend away is totally recommended, and it may even change your life. Whilst any of the below suggestions probably won't change your life, they might at least change your mood, your mindset or your day:
- a spa day
- a walk somewhere calming
- a shopping trip (even window shopping, but perhaps not your weekly supermarket dash)
- an hour with a book and a brew
- a solo swim
- a cinema/dinner date
- going for a scenic drive and singing along to your favourite music

Tape and glue and cracks of gold

♥ You're already enough, exactly as you are.

Do you know who you are?

You're already enough of everything you seek to be or everything you might falsely believe that you currently are not.

Do you know what has happened to you?

You've survived everything life has presented you with, and you have everything within you to survive another day. Believe in yourself enough to believe that you're worth the fight. Believe that you can continue to survive, until a tomorrow becomes a today where you feel able to heal and thrive and live the way you deserve to.

Do you want to live this way?

If your answer is no, or it's clouded in dissatisfaction, fear or doubt, there will always be a solution. There will always be an alternative perspective. There will always be a different mindset, a listening ear or a reassuring voice. There will always be a route to a source of light to penetrate whatever darkness you may currently be in, which will lead you to a place of acceptance, pride, and strength. There will always be a way to bring you back to yourself, to bring you power, and to enable you to repair and rebuild yourself from the inside out.

Mental health support services

Detailed below are various mental health support services that are accessible independently, dependent upon your need and circumstances. This list is not extensive and it was correct at the time of publication. It is intended to act as a means of providing options and opportunities to access services to support and maintain good mental health in times of crisis or vulnerability. That said, it is not my intention to endorse any one organisation through their inclusion within this book, or discredit any organisation omitted.

Should the need arise for you or someone you love, I hope this section proves useful.

If you, or someone you know, is in mental health crisis and requires immediate medical help:
Ring 999 to contact emergency services
Go to your nearest Accident and Emergency Department.

If it's not a medical emergency, but you still need urgent help:
Ring 111 for professional health advice 24/7, 365 days a year. You will receive guidance on where to access appropriate

health services.
Make an appointment with your GP.

Crisis and emotional support centres for everyone

The organisations detailed below provide emotional and crisis support for everyone affected by mental ill health.

Samaritans

Samaritans offer a non-judgemental and confidential service, in which you can talk through and about your feelings with empathy and impartiality. The number will not appear on your phone bill.
Phone: 116 123 (freephone, 24 hours a day, 7 days a week, 365 days a year)
Email: jo@samaritans.org
Website: www.samaritans.org

CALM (Campaign Against Living Miserably)

The CALM helpline answers a call every 59 seconds from people in distress, in emotional crisis or those who are suicidal. Through their website, they also offer a service directory of websites and services that offer support on a range of issues, from alcohol dependency, anxiety, depression, being a carer for someone

else, mental health support, wellbeing, and terminal illness.
Phone: 0800 58 58 58 (5pm – midnight, 365 days a year)
Website: https://www.thecalmzone.net/contact-us

SaneLine

SaneLine is a confidential support service for anyone aged 16 or over. It provides an out of hours service, offering support and information to people suffering with their emotional or mental health, or those dealing with issues like this from members of their family, friends, and carers. Their trained volunteers offer an empathetic and non-judgemental safe space to talk through any mental health related issues you or a loved one are encountering.
Phone: 0300 304 7000 (Local call charges apply, 4pm – 10pm, 7 days a week, 365 days a year)
Email: info@sane.org.uk
Website: https://www.sane.org.uk/who-we-are/contact-us

SHOUT

SHOUT is a free, confidential, 24/7 support service for anyone within the UK who's struggling to cope due to their mental health.

To start a conversation, **text the word 'SHOUT' to 85258.** Trained volunteers will respond to your messages, day or night, and will listen to whatever problem you're facing and whatever is on your mind. They aim to instil calm and enable you to support yourself going forward with a suggested plan for progression. Messages won't appear on your phone bill.

ANDYSMANCLUB

Since 2016, ANDYSMANCLUB has been offering peer-to-peer support to males aged 18 and over, via in-person support sessions at one of their 132 nationwide locations or via online support. Their service is used on a weekly basis by almost 2000 men. Its aim is to target #THATONEMAN who may be suffering in silence with their mental health. Non-judgemental conversation is always front and centre during weekly support sessions, so that future families can be spared the pain of losing a male family member. The Roberts family experienced this terrible scenario in 2016, when Andrew Roberts took his own life; none of his family were aware of what he was struggling against.

ANDYSMANCLUB offers a safe space where men can share their troubles and support one another to reduce the male suicide rate, one man at a time, with one conversation at a time. By visiting their website, you can find a free-to-attend support group in your local area, find more information or reach out to someone via email. The organisation is also active on social media sites LinkedIn, Facebook, Instagram and X (previously Twitter).

Website: https://andysmanclub.co.uk/
Email: info@andysmanclub.co.uk

The Hub of Hope
The Hub of Hope is the UK's leading mental health support database, bringing local, national, peer, community, charity, private, and NHS mental health support services together in one place. The website states: 'The services and support listed on the Hub of Hope are not only for when things become unbearable—a crisis point—they're also for those times when we notice we are starting to struggle, or when we need extra support as we start to emerge from a particularly difficult time.'

Website: https://hubofhope.co.uk

Mental health information helplines for everyone.

The following organisations provide advice and information on mental health; however, they cannot provide emotional or crisis support.

Mind Infoline

Mind Infoline provides information on types of mental health issues, where to get help, medication, and alternative treatments and advocacy.

Phone: 0300 123 3393 (Local call charges apply, 9am – 6pm, Monday – Friday)
Text: 86463

NHS: Self-help

This website provides a range of online material, covering issues such as bereavement, depression and low-mood, stress, anxiety, postnatal depression, panic, and social anxiety.
Website: https://web.ntw.nhs.uk/selfhelp

Action for Happiness

Founded in 2010, Action for Happiness is a registered charity based in the UK, whose ethos and mission is to support awareness of how to build happiness rituals into our everyday life on an individual basis. The organisation provides daily practical and mindful actions that people can take—through their website or app—to promote a happier and more positive way of life. It has an online community that discusses strategies towards creating and sustaining happiness, in addition to in-person talks and courses, school resources, and work-based training. It provides manageable strategies for understanding and implementing happiness to support the movement for a world where everyone can thrive rather than just survive.

Website: https://actionforhappiness.org/

Dear reader,

From the fact that you're holding this book in your hand, you've made one of my longest-held dreams come true. I've always had modest aspirations in life. I never imagined I would change the world or be rich or famous or be remembered by anyone other than those within my immediate circle. I never imagined that I would achieve anything beyond the ordinary. But this book has opened my eyes to so much, and it's been my greatest therapy and most significant means of giving back to the very world I'm trying to navigate. I've always loved to write. I've found comfort from putting my experiences and emotions to paper, and I've found strength in the healing this brought.

I've learned the hard way how short life is. I know this is a recycled cliché we all hear until the words cease to have meaning, but there really are no dress rehearsals or chances to come back and do it better next time around. There will be pain, overwhelming emotions, challenges, sacrifices, and moments that bring us to our knees. These represent the shade that frames the light—and there is light to be found. Light comes from others. It comes from moments, places, memories, and achievements. It comes fleetingly or regularly, depending on how receptive you are to it. Most importantly, it comes from within.

My hope, through this book, is that you begin to have deeper connections in your life with those you meet and love and that you take greater control of your life's direction and influences. I hope you see your journey and your progress as a daily milestone. I hope you listen to what it allows you to learn about yourself. I hope that you follow it, as it guides you to find your place in the world. Although there will always be shade waiting on the sidelines, never allow yourself to live or rest within the darkness or anyone else's shadow, or fade into the background. You have too much to give and you're too important to settle, to live small or to be defined by a bad day, a negative experience or anyone else's opinion.

Life isn't easy and tomorrow isn't promised. I hope you're able to embrace all that you are and move forwards, with just a little more hope, optimism, and self-love than you had before. I hope you remember that you're never as alone as you might feel at your lowest. I hope you remind yourself that you're already enough of all that you need to be. I'm not professionally qualified to change your life, but I am a person who has been broken, vulnerable, scared and scarred, and I want that pain to be worth something to someone. I've shared my experiences and my realisations in the hope that, if you're in a dark place, you can find your brighter horizon and your worth.

Thank you for investing your time in these pages. I really hope they've helped you in some way or resonated at some level. At the very least, I hope it has been an enjoyable way to pass the time.

Acknowledgements

This might seem an odd way to start, but I want to say thank you to everyone who has shaped me throughout my life. Thank you to those people who have forced me to become stronger and more emotionally resilient, and who, through their words and actions, sent me down a path I never chose to travel. This ultimately gave me the opportunity to grow, learn, hurt, and heal, and come out the other side stronger, kinder, and better.

I'm still travelling, but I've come to realise that this is the point of life. When we aren't travelling, we're standing still. This is fine and necessary if you're a tree, but people are made to be challenged and tested, and forced to adapt, change, and grow. That's how we're able to know, understand, and experience our limits and work to push beyond them. I've been to some version of hell, but, with determination and support, I brought myself back, and I'm now able to see the positive in those situations. You never know what you're capable of until you're forced to find out. I've always had the desire to write this book; life, people and experiences just gave me the reason.

This book would be no more than an inconceivable dream without my incredible, patient, supportive, and knowledgeable publisher, Diane. Like a fairy godmother, you allowed me to turn my ambition into a reality that surpassed both the stroke of midnight and all my expectations. Thank you will never be enough to express how much it means to hold this book in my hand and to have learned so many invaluable skills and lessons along the way. But I will say thank you from the bottom of my heart and I hope that's a start.

To my selfless and irreplaceable mum and dad, thank you for a lifetime of unconditional love, support and opportunities, and for being my biggest cheerleaders. All I've ever wanted to do is make a positive difference in the world and make you proud. I hope you know how grateful I am for everything you are, everything you do, and all that you've enabled me to become. From the bottom of my heart, I love and appreciate you more than you know.

To my nana and gran, I miss you every single day. When I see a toasted teacake, the Beano, a Hawaiian pizza, a host of golden daffodils or a pot of potpourri, I see you, my childhood, and my happiness. I see the brave, dignified, loving, inspirational women that you will always be to me. My love for you is immeasurable and the world was a better place for having you in it.

Emily, Michelle and Natalie, you are the most

inspirational, strong, positive women I know. I'm beyond proud of you and grateful for you. Life isn't always kind or fair, but you've looked it in the face and refused to back down or settle. I'm in awe of you and all that you are, and all that you continue to do.

I'm beyond grateful to every incredible friend I have for coming into my life, for making it infinitely better, and for never leaving. Thank you for seeing me as I am. Thank you for loving me unconditionally when I can't always love myself. Thank you for giving me incredible, life-affirming memories, more love, laughter and happiness than I ever thought possible, and the encouragement to never settle. Thank you for also giving me the greatest gift of being a godmother and an aunty. I can't tell you how grateful I am for you and your amazing children, and how much better my life is because of each one of you.

Jenna, Debbie, Katie, Natalie, Lucy, Debs, Parveen, Elliott, Laura, Sue, Nicola, Cath, Diana, Gill, Chris, Fid, Tara and Jimmy: I owe you more than I can express. You are irreplaceable, you're loved, and you are enough.

To every friend who has, throughout the years, believed in me enough to tell me that I should write a book, I'm so grateful for your encouragement, which lit the spark and spurred me on to this point. It may have taken me a while, but I got there in the end. I just hope it was worth the wait.

To all the children in my life I've been lucky enough to know, teach and love: you're all here for a reason and you're already enough of everything the world will attempt to judge you on. Never let it take your voice, your unique contribution, your precious awe and wonder, your strength or your happiness. You are enough, no matter what. I'm so proud of you and grateful for you. Thank you for the happiness you brought to my life and all the things you taught me; for allowing me to be a big kid–beyond what might be considered socially acceptable—and for how much better the world is because you exist and because you are who you are. For every hug we've shared, every deep conversation, all the laughter, each silly moment; for every Kodak moment, life-affirming moment, and so much more besides...thank you. You are loved.

References

ACEs – Adverse Childhood Experiences. Gloucestershire Healthy Living and Learning. (2017). https://www.ghll.org.uk/mental-health/aces---adverse-childhood-experiences

Action for Happiness - 10 Keys to Living Happier Lives. https://actionforhappiness.org/10-keys

Adverse Life Experiences (ACEs). https://lifechancetrust.org.uk/about/adverse-life-experiences-aces/

Brain Development: Meaning, Example and Psychology. https://www.studysmarter.co.uk/explanations/psychology/cognition/brain-development/

Fetal Brain Development Stages: When Does a Fetus Develop a Brain? (2020). https://flo.health/pregnancy/pregnancy-health/fetal-development/fetal-brain-development

Health and Social Care Committee. (2022). https://publications.parliament.uk/pa/cm5803/cmselect/cmhealth/114/report.html

How Much of Communication is Nonverbal? https://online.utpb.edu/about-us/articles/communication/how-much-of-communication-is-nonverbal/

How much blood gold in the human body?

(2021). https://esti.my/stem-facts/how-much-gold-could-be-found-in-a-human-body/

Mental Health Foundation. (2019). https://www.mentalhealth.org.uk/sites/default/files/2022-08/Body%20Image%20-%20How%20we%20think%20and%20feel%20about%20our%20bodies.pdf

Office for National Statistics. Census 2021. (2022). https://www.ons.gov.uk/peoplepopulationandcommunity/birthsdeathsandmarriages/ageing/articles/voicesofourageingpopulation/livinglongerlives

Parenting for Brain. Early Brain Development in Children. (2023) https://www.parentingforbrain.com/brain-development/

The Flea Experiment. https://possiblemind.co.uk/fleas-in-a-jar/

The Guardian. (2020). https://www.theguardian.com/money/2000/apr/18/workandcareers.pay

United Nations. https://www.un.org/en/global-issues/population

WHO. (2018). https://www.who.int/news-room/fact-sheets/detail/mental-health-strengthening-our-response